The New GP Survival Guide

for registrars, returners and all those new to UK General Practice

The New GP Survival Guide

for registrars, returners and all those new to UK General Practice

Siân Howell MB BS, MRCGP, DRCOG

General Practitioner, London

Emma Radcliffe MB BS, BSc (Hons), MRCGP, DRCOG

General Practitioner, London

and

Wendy Abrams MB BS, MRCGP, DRCOG

General Practitioner, London

Scion

A CIP catalogue record for this book is available from the British Library.

ISBN 1 904842 09 7

Scion Publishing Limited
Bloxham Mill, Barford Road, Bloxham, Oxfordshire OX15 4FF
www.scionpublishing.com

Important Note from the Publisher
The information contained within this book was obtained by Scion Publishing Limited from sources believed by us to be reliable. However, while every effort has been made to ensure its accuracy, no responsibility for loss or injury whatsoever occasioned to any person acting or refraining from action as a result of information contained herein can be accepted by the authors or publishers.

The reader should remember that medicine is a contantly evolving science and while the authors and publishers have ensured that all dosages, applications and practices are based on current indications, there may be specific practices which differ between communities. You should always follow the guidelines laid down by the manufacturers of specific products and the relevant authorities in the country in which you are practising.

Typeset by Phoenix Photosetting, Chatham, Kent, UK
Printed by Biddles Ltd, King's Lynn, UK, www.biddles.co.uk

Contents

Foreword

2005 is an excellent time for this new edition of the widely-commended *GP Registrar Survival Guide* to appear. It is, of course, an old Chinese curse to be fated to live in exciting times. And one could scarcely imagine any times more exciting than now to be working in general practice.

Think of how much change is presently affecting medical practice, and particularly primary care. GPs have a new contract, which could either drive standards up or morale down, depending on how successful we can be at preserving the core skills and values of clinical generalism. We have had the case of the appalling Dr Shipman, and are yet to see the full extent of change in our professional and regulatory environment that will flow from Dame Janet Smith's inquiry. There are major changes afoot in medical education, both in the early post-qualification period as the impact of *Modernising Medical Careers* brings more young doctors into practice for short placements, and in vocational training as the new Postgraduate Medical Education and Training Board comes on stream.

Not least, the demography of the general practice workforce is very different from what it was only a short time ago. Direct progression from vocational training to work as a full-time principal can no longer be assumed to be the norm. Many doctors now build portfolio careers, take career breaks, or gain other forms of experience before entering, or returning to, general practice. Many more find themselves working in the British NHS having trained overseas in very different systems of health care. As the change in this edition's title suggests, much of general practice is, if not 'new', at least unfamiliar to those who trained some time ago. And Britain's 'new GPs' are not necessarily all just graduating from their vocational training.

So there are an increasing number of doctors who will be grateful for a rapid induction into primary care as conducted in the United Kingdom. Such is the complexity of general practice that it would be very easy to be overwhelmed in the early days. Those of us who have been in practice for a while know, if we set aside the grumbling that doctors frequently enjoy, that general practice is the best job in the world. But in order to flourish and delight in this area of medicine, it is necessary first to survive. 'Sink or swim' is all very well as a slogan, but it's no way to treat expensively trained and highly skilled professionals! This book supplies a much-needed life jacket.

Clinical generalism is more complex and satisfying than is often appreciated. It is a great pleasure, therefore, to find that the authors manage to supply not just the minutiae of detail needed for survival, but also to convey a sense of the 'big picture' which will sustain the new GP in the difficult transition from learner to practitioner. I congratulate them on their achievement.

Roger Neighbour, MA DSc FRCP PRCGP
President, Royal College of General Practitioners
Bedmond, Herts
January 2005

Preface

The ethos, professionals and systems within primary care can be overwhelming to the newcomer. Whether you are a registrar, family doctor from another country or someone returning to general practice after a break, this book will aid your transition into UK primary care.

We have aimed to provide an up to date practical guide and resource tool for your daily work as a new GP.

This book is essentially the second edition of *The GP Registrar Survival Guide* published in 2002 and winner of a Society of Authors and Royal Society of Medicine award that year.

This new edition is still aimed primarily at the GP registrar but now also contains information for returners and doctors from abroad new to UK general practice.

Our advice is distilled from our experience and a wide variety of sources. We have tried to include everything we didn't know when we started in general practice but wished we had!

General practice is constantly developing and there are frequent changes in the organisation of the NHS, GP training and assessment. We have endeavoured to provide directions to where you can find the most up to date sources of information.

We hope you enjoy your experiences of general practice.

Good luck!

Siân Howell, Emma Radcliffe, Wendy Abrams
January 2005

Acknowledgements

We would like to thank the following people for their help: Margareth Attwood (National Office of Summative Assessment), Phil Bennett-Richards, Conor Byrne, Mike Callaghan, Philippa Cockman, Deborah Coleman, Allison Day, Ian Fryatt (Health Protection Agency), Bethan George, Paul Jakeman, Kate Nicholson, Gerard Panting (Medical Protection Society), Maggie Radcliffe, Philip Sawney and Anita Silk (Department of Work and Pensions), Pat Sharp, Geraldine Taylor, Anna Trigell, Rebecca Viney.

We would also like to acknowledge the help of: the Royal College of General Practitioners, the Department of Health, the British Medical Association, and the General Medical Council.

Abbreviations

A&E	Accident and Emergency
AA	Attendance allowance
AA	Alcoholics Anonymous
ACPC	Area Child Protection Committee
ADR	Adverse drug reaction
AHP	Allied health professional
AISMA	Association of Independent Specialist Medical Accountants
ALBs	Arms Length Bodies
ALS	Advanced life support
APMS	Alternative Provider of Medical Services
ASW	Approved social worker
ATLS	Advanced trauma life support
b.d.	Twice daily
BHS	British Hypertension Society
BJGP	British Journal of General Practice
BM Stix	Blood glucose monitoring sticks
BMA	British Medical Association
BMI	Body mass index
BMJ	British Medical Journal
BMS	Booking Management Service
BNF	British National Formulary
BP	Blood pressure
BPAS	British Pregnancy Advisory Service
CAS	Clinical Assessment Service
CD	Controlled drug
CHAI	Committee for Healthcare Audit and Inspection (Healthcare Commission)
CME	Continuing Medical Education
CMHT	Community mental health team
CMO	Chief Medical Officer
COC	Combined oral contraceptive pill
COGPED	Committee of General Practice Education Directors
CPD	Continuing professional development
CPN	Community psychiatric nurse
CPR	Cardiopulmonary resuscitation
CRP	C-reactive protein
CSCI	Commission for Social Care Inspection
CSM	Committee on Safety of Medicines

CVD	Cardiovascular disease
CXR	Chest X-ray
DCH	Diploma in Child Health
DDRB	Doctors and Dentists Review Body
DENs	Doctors' educational needs
DF118	Dihydrocodeine tartrate
DFFP	Diploma of the Faculty of Family Planning
DGM	Diploma in Geriatric Medicine
DHSSPSNI	Department of Health, Social Services and Public Safety, Northern Ireland
DLA	Disability living allowance
DMR	Diploma in Medical Rehabilitation
DN	District nurse
DOH	Department of Health
DPGPE	Director of Postgraduate General Practice Education
DRCOG	Diploma of the Royal College of Obstetricians and Gynaecologists
DTMH	Diploma in Tropical Medicine and Hygiene
DVLA	Driver and Vehicle Licensing Agency
DWP	Department for Work and Pensions
ECG	Electrocardiogram
ESR	Erythrocyte sedimentation rate
FBC	Full blood count
FFP	Faculty of Family Planning
FPA	Family Planning Association
FPHM	Faculty of Public Health Medicine
FPM	Faculty of Pharmaceutical Medicine
FRCGP	Fellow of the Royal College of General Practitioners
GMC	General Medical Council
GMS	General Medical Services
GP	General Practitioner
GPC	General Practitioners Committee
GPR	General Practitioner Registrar
GPwSI	GP with a specialist interest
GSL	General sales list medicine
HCA	Health Care Assistant
HPA	Health Protection Agency
HPE	Higher Professional Education
HRT	Hormone replacement therapy
HSA1	Form for termination of pregnancy
HSE	Health and Safety Executive
i.m.	Intramuscular
i.v.	Intravenous
IB	Incapacity benefit
ICAS	Independent Complaints Advocacy Service
INR	International normalised ratio
INT	Immediate and necessary treatment
IT	Information technology
IUCD	Intrauterine contraceptive device
JCPTGP	Joint Committee on Postgraduate Training for General Practice

LHCC	Local Health Care Cooperatives
LMC	Local Medical Committee
LNR	Leicester, Northamptonshire and Rutland
LoCIUT	Letter of competence in intrauterine techniques
MA	Maternity Allowance
MAP	Membership by assessment of performance (of the RCGP)
MAR	Medical Attendant's Report
MCQ	Multiple choice questionnaire
MDI	Metered dose inhaler
MHA	Mental Health Assessment
MHRA	Medicines and Healthcare Products Regulatory Agency
MIMS	Monthly index of medical specialities
MPIG	Minimum Practice Income Guarantee
MPO	Medical Protection Organisation
MRCGP	Member of the Royal College of General Practitioners
MSc	Master of Science
NASGP	National Association of Sessional GPs
NCAA	National Clinical Assessment Authority
ND	Notifiable Disease
NDDP	New Deal for Disabled People
NELH	National Electronic Library for Health
nGMS	New General Medical Services Contract (April 2004)
NHS	National Health Service
NHSIA	NHS Information Authority
NI	National Insurance
NICE	National Institute for Clinical Excellence
NILSI	NHS 'Institute of Learning, Skills and Innovation'
NIPPI	Northern Ireland Prescribing Prices Information
NOSA	National Office for Summative Assessment
NP	Nurse Practitioner
NPC	National Prescribing Centre
NPfIT	National Programme for Information Technology
NPMS	National Project Marking Schedule (summative assessment)
NPSA	National Patient Safety Agency
NSAID	Non-steroidal anti-inflammatory drug
NSF	National Service Framework
o.d.	Once daily
o.p.	One pack
OOH	Out of hours
OSCE	Objective structured clinical examination
OT	Occupational Therapist
OTC	Over the counter
P	Pharmacy medicine
p.o.	By mouth
p.r.	Rectally
p.r.n.	As required
p.v.	Vaginally
P45	Inland Revenue form documenting personal pay and tax details on leaving employment
PACT	Prescribing analysis and cost trend

PALS	Patient Advice and Liaison Service
PC	Performance criteria (for MRCGP video)
PCA	Personal capability assessment
PCC	Primary care centre
PCO	Primary care organisation
PCT	Primary care trust
PDP	Personal development plan
PEC	Professional Executive Committee
PEFR	Peak expiratory flow rate
PEP	Phased Evaluation Program
PHCT	Primary health care team
PILs	Patient information leaflets
PMETB	Postgraduate Medical Education Training Board
PMS	Personal medical services
PoM	Prescription only medicine
PPA	Prescription pricing authority
PPC	Prepayment certificate (for prescriptions)
PUNs	Patients' unmet needs
q.d.s.	Four times a day
QOF	Quality and outcome framework
RCGP	Royal College of General Practitioners
RCOG	Royal College of Obstetricians and Gynaecologists
RCP	Royal College of Physicians
RCPCH	Royal College of Paediatrics and Child Health
RCPsych	Royal College of Psychiatrists
RMO	Responsible Medical Officer
RSM	Royal Society of Medicine
RTA	Road Traffic Accident
s.c.	Subcutaneously
SHA	Strategic Health Authority
SIGN	Scottish Intercollegiate Guidelines Network
SMP	Statutory maternity pay
SOAP	Subjective, objective, assessment, plan
SOB	Shortness of breath
SPA	Scottish Prescribing Analysis
SSMG	Sure Start Maternity Grant
SSP	Statutory Sick Pay
t.d.s.	Three times a day
TCA	To come again
TCB	To come/call back
TCI	To come in
TFT	Thyroid function test
TOP	Termination of pregnancy
UTI	Urinary tract infection
VSO	Voluntary Service Overseas
VTR 1 and 2	Statements of satisfactory completion of registrar post (VTR 1) or educationally approved posts for GP training (VTR 2)
VTS	Vocational training scheme
WONCA	World Organisation of National Colleges, Academics and Academic Associations of General Practitioners/Family Physicians or World Organisation of Family Doctors

Chapter 1
Working in General Practice

INTRODUCTION

Despite the ever-changing and increasing role of the GP in the UK, the main 'raison d'être' has changed little over the last 50 years. General practice within the NHS provides personal and family health services to a small community over many years.

The GP is one of the first ports of entry into the NHS and has a gatekeeper and co-ordination role for secondary care and other services. GPs deal with new problems, long-term illnesses, emergency medical care as well as health promotion and the particular health needs of their community. Almost all GPs work within a multidisciplinary team*.

*See Chapter 2: Working in the team.

There are 40 000 GPs working in the UK as both principals and non-principals or sessional GPs. Over the last 10 years there has been a significant increase in the percentage of non-principals and a reduction in the number of single-handed GPs. An estimated 98% of the UK population is registered with a GP.

TYPES OF GP

Broadly speaking GPs are classified as either principals or sessional GPs (non-principal GPs) (*Box 1.1*). 'Principal' and 'partner' are often used synonymously, though not all principals work in partnership. Partnerships work within the framework of a legally binding 'Partnership Agreement'. The practice or partnership has a contract with the Primary Care Organisation (PCO) to take responsibility for a list of patients and the partners of that practice are then self-employed.

Sessional GPs are usually employed and paid by a practice or PCO.

GP CONTRACT

GP practices work under either a General Medical Services (GMS) contract, or Personal Medical Services (PMS) contract.

GMS

The new GP contract for GMS practices introduced in April 2004 is often denoted as nGMS for 'new'. Unlike the old contract, the nGMS contract is held with practices not individual doctors. A partnership must include one GP but can otherwise be made up of managers, nurses or other health professionals.

The nGMS contract has brought about enormous change in how GPs work. Its main thrust is rewarding quality of care, measured by quality indicators.

Money for practice infrastructure and running costs is provided in a global sum, dependent on weighted list size. Services are classified into essential, additional and enhanced (*Box 1.2*).

- Essential services - all practices are required to provide these

Box 1.1   Types of GP[a]

GP PRINCIPALS

Unrestricted principal
- provides a full range of General Medical Services (GMS) or Personal Medical Services (PMS)
- list not limited to any particular group of patients
- self-employed

Salaried Partner
- partnership status but with a guaranteed salaried income rather than a share of practice profits

SESSIONAL GPS

Salaried GPs (includes assistants and associates)
- employed by a practice, PCO or APMS (alternative provider of medical services)
- sessions may include peer support, clinical sessions in secondary care or research sessions
- some PCOs develop local schemes for salaried GPs

GP Locums
- contracted by practices to cover leave and other absence
- work on a short-term or occasional basis
- usually paid on a sessional basis
- self-employed

GP Retainers, GPs on Flexible Career Scheme and Returners
- work a prearranged limited number of sessions in a practice
- part of salary reimbursed by the PCO
- employing GPs responsible for continued training and support
- posts usually restricted in duration

- Additional services – all practices are expected to provide these unless they opt out, usually because of staffing problems
- Enhanced services – some are nationally directed and some locally directed when the practice will negotiate with their PCO on the terms and conditions to provide an agreed service

Further income is earned though the Quality and Outcomes Framework, QOF, which includes 76 quality indicators over 10 clinical domains (*Box 1.3*) and other organizational areas.

In order to maximize income from nGMS, practices must have up to date disease registers, run effective chronic disease management clinics, undertake patient questionnaires and keep up to date on administrative tasks, e.g. protocols and notes summarization.

nGMS also allows practices to opt out of out of hours work (OOH)*.

Practices have been given a 'Minimum Practice Income Guarantee' (MPIG) to ensure they did not lose out in the move from the old to the new contract. The MPIG is based on earnings under the old contract.

*See *Chapter 15: Out-of-hours work.*

PMS

Personal Medical Services pilots were introduced in 1998 when all other practices were working under the old GMS contract. The idea was to free

Box 1.3   nGMS Quality and Outcome Framework (QOF)

Clinical domains	Coronary heart disease
	Stroke
	Hypertension
	Hypothyroidism
	Diabetes
	Mental health
	COPD
	Asthma
	Epilepsy
	Cancer
Holistic Points	For the third lowest clinical domain to ensure work across the domains is recognised
Organisational domains	Records and information
	Communicating with patients
	Education and training
	Medicines management
	Clinical practice and management
Additional service domain	Cervical screening
	Child health surveillance
	Maternity services
	Contraceptive services
Patient experience domain	Patient survey
	Consultation length
Access	Access to a health professional within 24 hours and a doctor within 48 hours

practices from the administrative burden of claims under the old GMS and allows them to develop more 'personalised' services for their patient group, e.g. services for the homeless. Practices entered an individually negotiated contract with their PCO rather than the nationally negotiated old GMS contract which was outlined in the 'Red Book'. With the introduction of nGMS, PMS practices have access to the same funds for improving quality and outcome and enhanced services. They can also choose to opt out of OOH work. PMS practices are encouraged to use the nGMS quality and outcomes framework. However, there is the possibility of using local variations to address local circumstances, although any negotiated quality payments outside the nGMS framework must be evidence-based.

PCOs can also negotiate specialist PMS contracts with practices. These are directed primarily at vulnerable groups whose needs are not adequately met by other GMS or PMS providers, e.g. elders in care homes, people with learning disabilities, homeless persons.

Practice-based commissioning

From April 2005 practices can choose to hold an indicative budget for commissioning services from secondary care. This should incentivise practices to reduce referrals and increase services in primary care. Savings can be used to develop services within the practice.

Practices can group together to share indicative budgets, commissioning and any savings.

Non-NHS Income

GPs provide a number of services which are not GMS or PMS (*Box 1.4*) and are therefore not reimbursed by the NHS. Fees for these services are charged either to the patient or the third party requesting the GP service*.

*See *Chapter 12: Paperwork, certificates and benefits.*

Practices will be reimbursed for undergraduate teaching and for GP registrar training.

GPs may 'supplement' their income with work outside of the practice, as long as they have the agreement of their partners.

Non-NHS income may be pooled as general income for the practice or kept by the individual GP.

HOW THE PRACTICE IS ORGANISED

GP principals essentially run their own small businesses and so have great flexibility in how they organize themselves, their premises and the services they offer.

Each practice and each GP will have variable working patterns which develop over time and change to meet the needs of doctors, staff and patients[†].

†See *Chapter 4: Starting at the practice –* The practice timetable and rotas.

Running the practice

GP principals have the financial, management and staffing responsibilities of running a business but often have little or no formal training in business or management. They are also responsible for maintaining their surgery premises, which may be owned or leased.

While some GPs feel these responsibilities conflict with the basics of providing medical care, others like the control over their own working environment.

The relatively new salaried partner status was introduced to reduce some of this burden.

Professional managers are employed by most practices to avoid clinicians spending time on routine management tasks.

Box 1.4   Examples of non-NHS fees

Fee payable by patient
- Some travel vaccinations and vaccination certificates
- Medical examination for, e.g. HGV licence, pre-employment medical, fitness to drive
- Fitness to travel certificate
- Holiday cancellation letter
- Private health insurance claim form
- Statement of fact, e.g. confirmation of address, passport application forms (if you agree to sign them)
- Freedom from infection certificate

Fee payable by requesting organization
- Medical attendant's reports for life assurance and mortgages
- Police reports
- Legal reports
- Cremation forms
- Disabled parking badge
- Taxi card
- Notification of infectious disease

Other work within the practice
- Medical student teaching
- Registrar training
- Private patients (including tourists and non-UK nationals ineligible for NHS care).

Work undertaken outside the practice
- Police surgeon
- Work for the PCO
- Hospital clinical assistantships
- Private screening medicals
- Lectures and presentations

As a new GP or registrar, try to get a feel for what is involved in running a practice. This will be particularly useful if you are considering becoming a principal in the future.

The working day

Some practices start with commuter surgeries at 7am whilst others may have a later start and/or late evening surgeries. Many practices will close to patients completely between morning and evening surgery, with access to a doctor only in the case of emergencies. Larger practices may be more flexible in their opening hours.

*See *Chapter 15: Out of hours work.*

Out of hours* services cover from 6.30pm to 8am during the week, all weekends and bank holidays.

Appointments

Appointment types and systems vary but there are a few main types of appointments (*Box 1.5*). There is no ideal appointment system.

Ten minute appointment times and being able to see a GP within 48 hours and a health professional within 24 hours are quality markers in nGMS. Many practices now operate an appointment system under the 'Advanced Access' system. This involves measuring patient demand for appointments and ensuring this demand is met on a daily basis. It also involves 'shaping' demand by looking at skill mix in the team, use of telephone contacts with patients, etc. Ideally this prevents a backlog developing as 'today's work is done today'. Patients should always be able to pre-book appointments.

Box 1.5   Appointment types

Routine
- usually booked in advance with the patient's registered or preferred GP
- usually 10 minutes

Emergency
- usually available on the day, or at short notice
- short appointments for problems that cannot wait for a routine appointment
- may be with a Nurse Practitioner

Walk in
- Patients seen on a 'first come first served' basis

PARTNERSHIP AGREEMENTS

A partnership is a business arrangement and this is unstable if it is without a written partnership agreement. The agreement is usually drawn up by a lawyer and signed by all partners. It is particularly important in cases of disagreement or dispute (*Box 1.6*). Partnerships without an agreement are considered 'Partnerships at will' and are then governed by the 1890 Partnership Act. The BMA advises all practices to have an agreement and provides guidance on their website.

SOURCES AND FURTHER READING

1. Fry J. *General Practice – The Facts.* Radcliffe Medical Press, 1993.
2. Royal College of General Practitioners. *Profile of UK General Practitioners.* RCGP Information Sheet No.1 June 2004.
3. British Medical Association. *New GMS Contract 2003 – Investing in General Practice.* BMA, 2003.
4. British Medical Association. *Partnership Agreement Guidance.* General Practitioners Committee. BMA, 2004.
5. Oldham J. *Advanced Access booklet 2001.* National Primary Care Development Team; www.npdt.org
6. Department of Health; www.dh.gov.uk

Chapter 2
Working in the team

INTRODUCTION

GPs work in teams with other professionals, making up the primary health care team (PHCT) or multidisciplinary team (MDT).

Health professionals working in primary care may be employed by different agencies, making it confusing for the newcomer. Employers include GP practices, PCOs, local authorities, and community and hospital trusts. Teams may cover areas that differ from GP practice catchment areas, be based in your practice or another health centre.

Practices should regularly review their skill mix to ensure the most appropriate person has the most appropriate role. This may mean movement of tasks between doctors, nurses, health care assistants and clerical staff.

This chapter gives you an overview of most of the people you are likely to work with in general practice.

TEAMWORK

A skilled GP will be an effective team member, understanding their own and others' roles and responsibilities. Day to day conflict with GP colleagues, staff members or other PHCT members can be draining and undermine patient care. Despite this, there is little or no training for doctors on how to work as a good team member and good teamwork often seems to happen by chance. The contribution of all team members should be valued and the varying skills of members recognized.

Each professional retains individual responsibility and accountability for their work and though the GP often assumes leadership of the team this can be inappropriate if another team member is more skilled to lead on a particular issue.

Teams should have effective ways of communicating changes, e.g. a newsletter or full practice meeting. Meetings should have a clear structure, with an agenda, minutes and points for action. Conflict, which is part of all teams, should be aired early, in a supportive environment and not be allowed to fester. Clarifying the conflict in writing, e.g. on a board, may help the whole team approach the problem rather than polarizing those in conflict.

It is a very rare GP practice that has not experienced some type of conflict. You may find you don't get on with a member of the team. Recognize this as a learning opportunity; reflect on your own role, it may happen again in teams you work with in the future. Registrars could use an experience of conflict as a basis for a tutorial.

Keep documentation of any conflict management you have been involved in for your appraisal folder*.

*See *Chapter 20: Appraisal and revalidation.*

THE CORE PRIMARY HEALTH CARE TEAM

This embodies the clinical and administrative staff (*Box 2.1*) working together for the care of a practice population.

GP practices usually employ clinical and administrative in-house staff whereas PCOs employ community medical staff, mainly district nurses, health visitors and midwives. These Allied Health Professionals (AHPs) may be based in your surgery premises but 'shared' with other practices.

Box 2.1   The core primary health care team

GPs
Practice nurses
District nurses
Health visitors
Practice manager
Administrative staff

STAFF EMPLOYED BY GP PRACTICES

Nursing staff

Practice nurse

Most practices employ a practice nurse, some of whom will hold a practice nurse diploma (*Box 2.2*). The practice retains a responsibility for their training, and supervision. Some nurses have an extended role in prescribing. The PCO will usually have a Practice Nurse coordinator who has a support, training and liaison role.

Chronic disease management by practice nurses is essential in reaching quality targets*.

*See Chapter 1: Working in general practice.

Nurse practitioner

Nurse practitioners (NPs) take on more responsibility than practice nurses, with an obvious overlap, and they will hold or be working towards a nurse practitioner degree. They work more autonomously, may have a role in prescribing, give telephone advice and may also undertake home visits. They may triage emergency cases and see uncomplicated presentations in the surgery. Some NPs have their own patient case loads, organise investigations and refer on to secondary care. They may also work with GPs to provide OOH care†.

†See Chapter 15: Out of hours work.

Box 2.2   Within the practice nurse remit

Health checks
- new patient registration
- long term illness, e.g. diabetes
- elderly health
- travel advice

Practical procedures
- blood pressure
- blood tests
- dressing and wound care
- spirometry
- cervical smears
- suture removal
- immunisations
- ear syringing
- diaphragm and cap fitting

Health promotion
- contraception
- diet
- exercise
- smoking
- alcohol
- sexual health

Health care assistant

HCAs may be employed to support and work within the nursing team. PCOs run courses for HCAs and there are NVQ qualifications. Their roles may include new patient checks, phlebotomy, smoking cessation advice, BP checks and other nursing support.

Administrative staff

Practice manager

The practice manager is responsible for the overall running of the practice, management of staff and practice finances, day-to-day administration, liaison with outside agencies and any problems arising. An experienced practice manager may take the practice lead on audit, clinical governance and strategic planning. Your practice manager will usually organize your pay, pension, contract and leave*.

See Chapter 4: Starting at the practice.

There are diplomas in practice management and many regions run part-time local training but these are not mandatory. Practice managers come from a variety of career backgrounds including management and nursing.

Receptionists

The receptionist remit includes dealing with patient requests, appointments, prescriptions and medical records as well as other administrative tasks; they should never give clinical advice. Although some courses exist, most receptionists will have no particular training for what can be a complex and stressful job.

Long-serving receptionists can be a mine of useful information on the who's who of patients, including the local 'celebrities'.

Support the reception team by reinforcing to patients the practice policies, e.g. the use of emergency appointments and requests for repeat prescriptions, particularly where you know patients have been difficult at reception. If a patient has been rude to a receptionist then ask them to apologize directly and document the episode in the patient's notes.

Secretary

Most practices have secretaries who type referral letters, arrange faxes, chase up appointments and deal with other administrative or IT tasks. They may have a thorough knowledge of local consultants, private specialists, agencies and waiting times.

Other administrative staff

Practices may employ administrators to assist the practice manager; clerks for filing, photocopying, ordering leaflets, general office duties and staff with IT skills for inputting clinical information, organising searches and audit.

COMMUNITY CLINICAL TEAM

District nurses

District nurses, also known as community nurses, have a community nursing qualification and are involved in the care of housebound patients. They manage long-term disability and chronic illness (*Box 2.3*) but do not provide personal care such as washing, dressing and feeding.

Liaise with district nurses before and after visiting any housebound patients known to them*. Most practices hold regular meetings with the district nurse team to review and revise management plans for shared patients.

*See *Chapter 14: Home visits – An approach to visiting.*

Box 2.3　District nursing

- Ulcer and wound care
- Administering medication and ensuring drug concordance/compliance
- Continence assessments and organizing pads, catheter care and commodes
- Monitoring chronic diseases
- Palliative care

Health visitors

Health visitors are responsible for health promotion and prevention, working with individuals, families and groups. The majority of their work is with children aged 10 days to 5 years and a good health visitor is a mine of useful information on childcare and rearing.

*See Chapter 22: Clinical issues with legal stipulations – Child protection.

They undertake much of the child development and screening work and monitor families at risk. They can provide support to families who are having difficulties coping*.

Community midwives

Community midwives see women for antenatal care in the community, either in clinics or at the woman's home, and liaise with the GP and hospital obstetricians involved in the woman's shared care. They can work independently in uncomplicated cases but must request a doctor's opinion when complications arise.

They attend women for home births. They will visit all mothers and babies at home regularly for the first 10 days after delivery, after which the health visitor takes over.

GP registrars should sit in on a midwife-led antenatal clinic.

Community physiotherapists

Community physiotherapists provide physiotherapy at home to patients with chronic respiratory problems, stroke rehabilitation and other immobilising conditions. Some practices have a physiotherapist in the practice.

Community mental health teams

All patients with a significant mental health problem living in the community should have a named worker from the Community Mental Health Team

(CMHT). The teams include community psychiatric nurses (CPNs), social workers, occupational therapists, psychologists and psychiatrists working together in a community setting.

A key worker from the CMHT will see their clients regularly for support and counselling. They should let the client's GP know when problems arise and when medication needs changing. They may avert admissions with increased community support for their clients experiencing difficulties.

Community paediatric team

Community paediatric teams (*Box 2.4*) work with children with development and speech delay, behavioural and emotional problems. They accept referrals from GPs, school nurses and health visitors.

Community paediatricians co-ordinate local services for immunisations, child health surveillance and children with special needs. They may be involved in child protection procedures* and run special immunisation clinics for children with egg allergy or previous immunisation reactions.

*See *Chapter 22: Clinical issues with legal stipulations* – Child protection.

Box 2.4   Community paediatric team

- Community paediatrician
- Physiotherapists
- Occupational therapists
- Speech therapists
- Audiology services
- Psychologists
- Child psychiatrists
- Paediatric nurses

Community intermediate care team

Intermediate care teams work between primary and secondary care and aim to support patients in their homes after hospital discharge, hopefully reducing their in-patient stay. They work with patients to try and prevent admission to hospital. This may involve some nursing, physiotherapy or simply domestic input for elderly patients who are unwell.

Community palliative care team

These multidisciplinary teams work from hospitals or hospices to provide care to terminally ill patients. They offer expert nursing and medical support and can gain prompt access to social services and occupational therapy†.

†See *Chapter 14: Home visits* – Terminally ill patients.

Community matrons

This relatively new group of nurses has been introduced as a result of the NHS Improvement Plan (2004) to produce personalized care packages for patients with long term illness living in the community. The aim is to improve care and prevent hospital admissions.

Community occupational therapists

OTs help patients overcome and live with disability. They have degree level training and may be employed by PCOs, hospital trusts or local authorities. They can arrange amendments for the home, e.g. rails and ramps. OTs may work within a community team, e.g. mental health and palliative care.

Other sessional workers

A variety of professional and voluntary workers (*Box 2.5*) may do regular or occasional sessions in your practice.

Box 2.5   Health professionals doing sessional work

Professions allied to medicine
- Counsellors and clinical psychologists
- Phlebotomists
- Hospital consultants
- Physiotherapists
- Occupational therapists
- Specialist nurses, e.g. continence nurse, ulcer nurse, colostomy advisor
- Podiatrist
- Dietician
- Alcohol and drug workers

Social and benefits
- Citizen's advice bureau worker
- Benefits advisor
- Age-concern worker
- Social worker

LOCAL AUTHORITY STAFF

Local authorities employ the staff involved in social care and housing: social workers, home help and local authority housing staff and wardens.

Social workers

Social workers have a degree or diploma in social work. They will take referrals from the clients or their carers and GPs.

A duty social worker is on-call 24 hours a day for emergencies mostly relating to mental health sections and child protection. Each speciality team will also have a duty social worker taking the referrals for that day.

Social services for the elderly

Refer patients to arrange assessments for services (*Box 2.6*).

Social services may be able to provide increased packages of care at short notice. This is particularly useful for elderly patients who become unwell and may prevent a hospital admission.

Box 2.6   Social services for the elderly

- Home help
- Meals on wheels
- Personal care
- Night sitters
- Personal alarms
- Day-centre attendance
- Assessments for possible residential care (local authority or private)

Mental health social services

Most patients with a significant mental health problem living in the community will have a named social worker, often working in a community mental health team with CPNs. They will provide general support and counselling as well as helping with social, benefit and housing needs. Approved social workers are key players in arranging 'sections'*.

*See *Chapter 22: Clinical issues with legal stipulations* – The Mental Health Act and the acutely mentally ill patient.

Children and families social services

Children and families social workers have a statutory duty to investigate cases where a child is at risk[†]. There is often both stigma and fear attached to a referral to social services so try to emphasize their supportive role and the benefit of their early involvement when discussing referral with families.

†See *Chapter 22: Clinical issues with legal stipulations* – Child protection.

OTHER COMMUNITY HEALTH PROFESSIONALS

All of the following are available on the high street as a private service. Some may provide an NHS funded service.

Pharmacists

You will have daily interactions with your local pharmacists especially over prescribing queries. There is a big push for greater involvement of pharmacists in medication reviews and general medicines management, with improved communications with IT links to practices.

Your PCO may employ pharmacists to advise on local prescribing initiatives, audit and evidence-based prescribing*.

*See *Chapter 8: Prescribing –* Drug information sources.

Podiatrists

Hospitals and PCOs employ podiatrists (chiropodists) to provide foot care, usually for the elderly and patients with diabetes, as well as those with other clinical needs, e.g. in-growing toenails. Private high street chiropodists cater for everybody else.

Opticians

High street opticians offer free eye checks to some patients, e.g. family history of glaucoma. Patients who work on VDUs should have regular eye checks paid for by their employer

Dentists

Community dentists are usually self-employed but some may work for PCOs. High street dentists offer a private or NHS service or a combination of the two. They are reimbursed for NHS dental care provided to patients exempt from charges. All dentists should provide an OOH service to their patients for dental emergencies so this should not fall to GPs.

GPs are occasionally asked to prescribe prophylactic antibiotics to patients at risk from endocarditis before dental treatment, and for details of medical conditions that may affect their dental treatment. Dentists can, however, prescribe antibiotics. Hospital dental departments deal with specialist dental needs.

SOURCES AND FURTHER READING

1. RCGP. *The Primary Health Care Team,* Information Sheet No. 21, October 2003.
2. Department of Health. *The NHS Improvement Plan*, 2004.

Chapter 3
Working in the wider health service

INTRODUCTION

As a new GP you need to be aware of the many agencies that will affect your working life. It's worth trying to keep abreast of the changes in health care organization, education and medical politics for your general information and the MRCGP exam. This can be overwhelming as just as you manage to get a grasp on things, it will all seem to change again.

This chapter aims to simplify things for you by giving you details of the main agencies you need to know about. Keep up to date with changes by reading the GP press and Department of Health publications and accessing their websites.

GPs do have fora for political representation and these can influence the directives from on high. GP registrars can get involved through the GP Registrars Subcommittee of the General Practitioners Committee (GPC) of the BMA and your faculty office of the Royal College of General Practitioners (RCGP) (see below).

Some of the organizations discussed cover all UK countries, some just England, or England and Wales. Check through your country's health websites for variations in organizations and their remit.

PROFESSIONAL

The General Medical Council

This national regulatory body acts as the watchdog for professional standards for doctors working in the UK. It both sets and oversees standards for medical education and professional practice. The main job of the General Medical Council (GMC) is to protect the public – rather than doctors. It is self-financing through the annual retention fee.

The GMC has four main functions in law:

- keeping up to date registers of qualified doctors
- fostering good medical practice
- promoting high standards of medical education
- dealing firmly and fairly with doctors whose fitness to practice is in doubt

Doctors must be registered with the GMC to practice medicine in the UK. The GMC is introducing a licence to practice linked to revalidation to ensure doctors remain up to date and fit to practice*.

*See Chapter 20: Appraisal and revalidation.

The GMC has the power to remove doctors from the register temporarily or permanently and to revoke their licence to practice medicine in the UK.

The GMCs advice to doctors on good professional conduct is formalized in its set of guidance booklets, *Good Medical Practice*, and all doctors receive regular updates of these.

The GMC has recently reformed and streamlined its fitness to practice procedures and full details are available on their website.

SERVICE RELATED

Organizational

Organization of the NHS

The structure and management of the NHS varies between UK countries and undergoes constant change (*Box 3.1*).

In England, the Department of Health sets the overall direction of the NHS and sets national standards. Strategic health authorities plan health services in their area and have a responsibility to ensure that quality care is provided and that national plans are integrated into local services. Local services are commissioned by Primary Care Trusts (PCTs), from Hospital Trusts, community services, including general practice and the private sector.

Some hospital trusts can choose to be NHS Foundation Trusts, independent organizations run by locally elected Governors. These foundation trusts are freed from central control but regularly audited to ensure good quality care (see *Healthcare Commission* below).

In Wales, Local Health Boards are responsible via regional offices to the Welsh Assembly. They commission services from hospitals, GPs and other community services to provide health care in their area.

In Scotland, the Scottish Executive Health Department oversees the work of health boards, which are responsible for planning local health services and for self-governing NHS Trusts and Community Health Partnerships, which provide the services.

In Northern Ireland, Area Health and Social Services Boards assess health needs locally and contract services to meet these needs. Health and Social

---

Box 3.1   Organization of the NHS

England	Wales	Scotland	N.Ireland
The Department of Health	NHS Office of the National Assembly	Scottish Executive Health Department	Department of Health, Social Services and Public Safety
www.dh.gov.uk	www.wales.nhs.uk	www.show.scot.nhs.uk	www.dhsspsni.gov.uk
Strategic Health Authorities	Local Health Boards	Health Boards	Health and Social Services Boards
NHS Trusts – primary care, hospital, foundation, care, mental health, ambulance	NHS Trusts – hospital, community and primary care, and local health groups	NHS Trusts – hospital, community and primary care and local health care co-operatives	Health and Social Services Trusts

Services Trusts and Local Health and Social Care Groups are the local providers of services and control their own budgets.

There are some special health authorities that are UK wide, e.g. transplant services and special hospitals.

Arm's length bodies (ALBs) (*Box 3.2*) is the term used for the independent organizations, sponsored by the Department of Health to undertake executive functions.

Box 3.2 Arms length bodies

- The National and Primary Care Trust Development Programme
- The National Primary Care Development Team
- The NHS Pensions Agency
- The Health Protection Agency
- NHS Estates
- The Medicines and Healthcare Products Regulatory Agency

Primary Care Organisations

The term PCO can usually be taken to mean PCTs in England, Primary Care Groups in Wales, Health and Social Services Trusts in Northern Ireland and Primary Care NHS Trusts in Scotland.

Primary Care Trusts

PCTs in England receive 80% of NHS funding (2004). They are locally based and both deliver and commission services. Leadership is shared by the Trust Board and the Professional Executive Committee (PEC) which represent doctors, allied health professionals, patients and management. The PCT must ensure that all health services are provided in their area, including primary care, hospital services, mental health and community health services. The local Strategic Health Authority monitors their work. The PCT will negotiate contracts with individual practices and reimburse them for services provided. PCTs should involve clinicians in management decisions and there are opportunities for GPs to join committees and working groups.

Check out your PCT website for up to date information on their management structure and current priorities.

Quality assurance

Healthcare Commission

The Commission for Healthcare Audit and Inspection (CHAI), shortened to the Healthcare Commission, took over from CHI (Commission for Health Improvement) in 2004.

It is an independent inspection body for all NHS, private and voluntary health services with a remit to inspect, inform and improve. It reviews performance of bodies and publishes results aiming to improve patient choice. It is the organization that gives healthcare organizations their stars. It has a complaints service for patients and carers unhappy with how their complaints have been dealt with locally. From 2004 it took on the responsibility for work done by the Mental Health Act Commission which was closed.

National Patient Safety Agency

The NPSA was set up in July 2001 following the report of the then Chief Medical Officer called *An Organisation with a Memory*. The report proposed developing a culture of openness and safety consciousness through all NHS organizations and to improve patient safety by reducing the risk of harm through error. Their remit is to collect and analyze data, learn lessons and produce solutions for all sectors of the NHS.

National Clinical Assessment Authority

Part of the NPSA, the National Clinical Assessment Authority (NCAA) addresses concerns about the performance of doctors. They will undertake assessments of doctors when local procedures have not been effective or are not appropriate. In primary care they provide expert advice to PCOs on local procedures and individual cases. Assessments are formative, educational rather than summative (pass/fail), and make recommendations to the referring organization. The NCAA do not assess fitness to practice, which is done by the GMC. Any serious concerns raised from their assessment will be passed on to the referring organization. GPs registrars can only be referred to the NCAA by their Deanery.

Medicines and Healthcare Products Regulatory Agency

This Executive Agency of the Department of Health was formed in 2003 from the merging of the Medicines Control Agency (MCA) and the Medical Devices Agency (MDA). The remit of the MHRA is to ensure the safety of drugs and medical devices.

Committee on Safety of Medicines

This independent committee advises the MHRA on whether new products should be granted marketing authorization and monitors the safety of marketed medicines. It operates the 'yellow card' system for suspected adverse drug reactions, and you should fill one of these in (available in the back of your *BNF*) if you suspect an adverse drug reaction. They are responsible for licensing medicines and regulating medical devices. Their web pages are available via the MHRA website.

Health Protection Agency

This agency for England and Wales works to integrate services to reduce the impact of infectious diseases, poisons, chemicals and biological and radiation hazards. The HPA brings together the old Public Health Laboratory Service, Centre for Applied Microbiology and Research, National Poisons Information Service and NHS staff responsible for infectious disease control and emergency planning. They work to inform health professionals and the public and provide a rapid response to health protection emergencies. Local action is taken by the Directors of Public Health in the PCOs and SHAs.

Clinical services

National Institute for Clinical Excellence

NICE produces guidance for use by professionals and the public in England and Wales:

● on the use of existing medicines and treatments
● through clinical guidelines for specific conditions and diseases
● on the use of interventional procedures for diagnosis and treatments

Hopefully, NICE guidance will reduce the postcode lottery of NHS treatment. NICE guidance is circulated to all doctors on a regular basis and is also available on the website.

NHS Direct

*See *Chapter 15: Out of hours work*.

This 24 hour nurse-led telephone service in England and Wales (Scotland has a similar system with NHS-24) offers advice on personal health issues and information on accessing NHS services. NHS Direct has developed a role in some areas in working with OOHs* and will be the first contact for all OOH contacts from 2006.

NHS Walk-in Centres

Introduced in 1999 in various sites in England, these centres provide a nurse-led service to 'complement and supplement' GP services. Their remit is to provide face-to-face advice on minor illness and injuries and health promotion issues. They are open during the day, evenings and weekends. Like NHS Direct some PCTs have incorporated the walk-in centres with primary care OOH provision.

Patient services

Patient Advice and Liaison Service

Each trust, PCO and hospital has a PALS to help patients and their families access local services and support them if they have complaints. They provide feedback to the Trust on system failures and gaps in service. Search your local trust website for details of their PALS.

POLITICAL

British Medical Association

As the professional association and union for UK doctors, the BMA lobbies government on issues affecting doctors via numerous standing committees.

Eighty per cent of UK doctors are members. Benefits include the weekly *British Medical Journal*, access to Medline and an excellent library. Advice on working practices, disputes, entitlements and staffing issues are available to members though the regional offices.

General Practitioner Committee

As the sole negotiating body for GPs with the Department of Health, this standing committee of the BMA represents all GPs working in the NHS in England. There are separate Welsh and Scottish committees. The Northern Ireland Committee is autonomous of the GPC but works closely with it.

GP Registrars Subcommittee of the GPC

This subcommittee represents GPs in training both in hospital and general practice posts. Regional registrars' committees elect representatives to the subcommittee which is involved in policy nationally and in advising on terms of service and educational issues. It produces a newsletter and updated guidance on registrars' employment, contract and salary issues*. A list of local representatives and committees is available from the BMA. Under trade union law, employers must allow paid leave for representatives to attend meetings. If you get involved, seek your trainer's approval for such leave.

*See *Chapter 5: Contract and finances.*

Local Medical Committee

Your LMC is made up of local elected GPs who meet monthly to discuss and represent GPs' interests and working practices in your PCT area. LMC representatives meet annually at a national conference and approved motions are passed to the GPC for implementation. Each LMC is funded by subscriptions from local GPs.

National Association of Sessional GPs

Previously called the National Association of Non-Principals (NANP) and affiliated to the BMA, the NASGP represents the estimated 7500 salaried or freelance GPs in the UK. It aims to ensure representation of sessional GPs on

LMCs and the GPC. They lobby for employment and pension rights and the inclusion of non-principals in educational initiatives and information distribution. They produce a regular newsletter and put non-principals in touch with each other for local support and study groups*. They have a useful website and hold a regular conference.

*See Chapter 23: Career options for general practitioners.

EDUCATIONAL

Joint Committee on Postgraduate Training for General Practice / Postgraduate Medical Education and Training Board

At the time of going to press the JCPTGP was still responsible for postgraduate training in general practice. The JCPTGP requirements are available on their website and in their very useful publication *A Guide to Certification*.

The PMETB is due to start taking over this role from late 2005. Check their website for the most up to date information on training issues.

Deaneries

Postgraduate medical and dental training is delivered regionally through the deaneries. The GP section of the deanery organizes GP vocational training schemes (VTS), training of GP trainers and the employment and training of retainers, returners and EU GPs from fast-track training.

GP training is led by the Postgraduate Director of General Practice Education (usually known as the Dean) and a group of directors with support staff. Each deanery has a website with up to date training schedules, courses and publications relevant to training.

Royal College of General Practitioners

The RCGP acts as the voice of GPs on education, training, research and standards. It has faculties throughout the UK that organize educational and social events.

†See Chapter 18: The MRCGP exam.

Membership of the college is via the MRCGP exam[†] or membership by assessment of performance (MAP). Associate membership is available to those in training or who do not wish to sit the exam but want to support the college. All GP registrars are encouraged to join at a reduced subscription. Fellowship of the college (FRCGP) is awarded to members who have made significant contributions to the college or general practice development.

Benefits of membership include the monthly *British Journal of General Practice*, discounts on RCGP publications and benefits of the local faculties. Hotel and conference accommodation is available in London. The college also offers educational bursaries specifically for GPs in training and Education Fellowships for GPs carrying out research in GP settings.

Academic Departments of General Practice and Primary Care

Each medical school has a Department of General Practice or Primary Care that has a responsibility for undergraduate and postgraduate teaching as well as research. They may undertake research locally and nationally and in conjunction with other specialty departments*.

*See *Chapter 23: Career options for general practitioners –* Academic posts.

Royal Society of Medicine

Based in central London, the RSM provides a forum for education and exchange of ideas in all medical fields. It has an excellent GP section with regular academic meetings and a superb library. It also has a good restaurant and inexpensive accommodation for members.

NHS Institute of Learning, Skills and Innovation

The NILSI was introduced in 2004 to replace the work of the NHS University and Modernisation Agency. Its remit is to lead on NHS innovation, learning and leadership.

GP INTERNATIONAL

WONCA – World Organization of Family Doctors

WONCA actually stands for the rather long-winded World Organization of National Colleges, Academics and Academic Associations of General Practitioners/Family Physicians. This international organization has group and individual membership and holds three-yearly global conferences. They have official relations and work in collaboration with the World Health Organization as a non-government organization. Their meetings are a good way to meet primary care doctors from all around the world.

OTHER ORGANISATIONS

National Programme for IT

This agency (the NPfIT) has the remit to develop, procure and implement a modern IT infrastructure for all NHS organizations by 2010. It is a time-limited programme and will close on completion.

NHS Confederation

This is a UK-wide organization of NHS organizations. It works to influence policy and connect health leaders. It has an annual conference, regional events and policy development seminars. It advises the DOH directly.

SOURCES AND FURTHER READING

1. GMC. *A Licence to Practice and Revalidation.* April 2003.
2. RCGP. *The Structure of the NHS,* Information Sheet. November 2004.
3. Department of Health, www.dh.gov.uk
4. NHS information, www.nhs.uk
5. NHS Wales, www.wales.nhs.uk
6. Department of Health and Social Security Northern Ireland, www.dhsspsni.gov.uk
7. NHS Scotland, www.show.scot.nhs.uk
8. NHS Confederation, www.nhsconfed.webhoster.co.uk
9. Healthcare Commission, www.chai.org.uk
10. National Patient Safety Agency, www.npsa.nhs.uk
11. National Clinical Assessment Authority, www.ncaa.nhs.uk
12. Medicines and Healthcare Products Regulatory Agency, www.mhra.gov.uk
13. Health Protection Agency, www.hpa.org.uk
14. National Institute of Clinical Excellence, www.nice.org.uk
15. NHS Direct, www.nhsdirect.nhs.uk
16. British Medical Association, www.bma.org.uk
17. Royal College of General Practitioners, www.rcgp.org.uk
18. Royal Society of Medicine, www.roysocmed.ac.uk
19. NHS University, www.nhsu.nhs.uk
20. WONCA, www.globalfamilydoctor.com
21. Joint Committee on Postgraduate Training for General Practice, www.jcptgp.org.uk
22. Postgraduate Medical Education and Training Board, www.pmetb.org.uk
23. NHS Information Authority, www.nhsia.nhs.uk
24. National Programme for Information Technology, www.npfit.nhs.uk

Chapter 4
Starting at the practice

INTRODUCTION

All new GPs should have a time-tabled introduction to a new practice; this may be a few weeks long for GP registrars, but shorter for trained GPs.

Use your induction time to:

1. orientate yourself in the practice and sit in with colleagues
2. establish your weekly timetable
3. get ready for consulting and visiting*
4. organise your personal administration for employment purposes†
5. registrars should start planning their educational year‡

*See *Chapter 6: Practical preparations for clinical work.*

†See below and *Chapter 5: Contract and finances.*

‡See *Chapter 16: Educational aspects of the GP registrar year.*

PRACTICE TOUR

**See *Chapter 2: Working in the team.*

Your first day should include a practice tour and introduction to all team members**.

See *Box 4.1* for a checklist of what should be covered in the ideal practice tour.

PERSONAL ADMINISTRATION

We have included a checklist of what you need to bring or get hold of when starting in a new post; the practice manager should help you with this (*Box 4.2*).

Medical Performers List

In order to provide GP services, either GMS or PMS, all GPs, including GPRs, must be on the Performers List of the PCO. This list, but not all submitted personal details, is available to the public. A GP can only be on one PCO list at any one time but once on one list is able to work in the region covered by another PCO within the same UK country.

Application to your PCO involves completion of a form, two satisfactory medical references and submission of supporting documentation (see *Box 4.3*) including a criminal record check. Guidance for accessing this should be provided on the application form. As GPRs don't yet have a vocational training certificate they need to submit their trainer's details instead. Provided your application is underway you can work as a GPR for 2 months whilst the paperwork is processed.

Get your practice manager to help you out with all of this.

Box 4.1 Practice tour

Clinical
Treatment room
Specimen collection
Resuscitation equipment and training on use
Clinical supplies and who is responsible for restocking
Drug cupboard and controlled drugs – procedure for restocking,
    administration and disposal
Vaccines

Administrative
Trays for post, filing, scanning, colleagues
Message/visit books
Dictaphone and tapes
Stationery supplies
Photocopier
Shredding/recycling

Refreshment
Coffee and tea facilities
Staff toilets and lockers

Communications
Phone system
Contact system for duty doctor
E-mail
Fax
Patient call system

Building related
Parking
Security codes
Practice alarm system procedure
Locking up procedure

Health and safety
Panic alarm system
Health and safety policy
Fire drill and escape routes
Accident book
Sharps injury protocol

Box 4.2   Personal administration checklist

Professional certificates
GMC
Medical Protection Organisation (MPO)
Evidence of hepatitis B immunity
JCPTGP/PMETB certificate or equivalent unless starting as a registrar

Employment and salary
Contract
Bank details for receiving salary
P45
Birth certificate/passport (for pension purposes)
Staff transfer form from previous post
Medical Performers List
Enhanced criminal record certificate
Inform vehicle insurer of intention to use vehicle for business purposes

Education and training requirements for registrars
National training number
Current guidance on:
   JCPTGP/PMETB certification
   Summative assessment
   MRCGP regulations

Box 4.3   Documentation for PCO Medical Performers List application

- Birth certificate or passport for UK citizens
- Passport only for non-UK citizens
- Vocational Training Certificate (or trainer's details for GPR)
- GMC Registration Certificate
- Evidence of membership of a recognised medical protection organization
- Medical qualifications certificates
- Enhanced criminal record check

YOUR TIMETABLE

Your timetable should include a basic weekly timetable, your visiting schedule, duty doctor sessions, the practice-based tutorial and VTS release course for registrars. Antenatal, well-baby and other specialist clinics are a useful part of registrar training.

Include practice and postgraduate centre meetings in your timetable and identify a time for paperwork and clinical queries. Registrars should have protected time for tutorials (see *Box 4.4*) and returners may have protected clinical supervision time.

If you are a registrar and your regular sessions don't coincide exactly with your trainer, find out who will be supervising you in their absence.

GPRs also need to work out their OOH commitment and supervision for this*.

*See *Chapter 15: Out of hours work.*

Box 4.4   Basic GP registrar timetable

Full-time registrar:
- six or seven clinical sessions including special clinics, e.g. antenatal
- Tutorial
- VTS release course
- Half day
- Protected time for summative assessment obligations
- Out of hours work

PRACTICE TIMETABLE AND ROTAS

Find out how the overall practice timetable works. Identify the times of GP and nurse surgeries, book-in-advance, 'on the day' and urgent appointments, and practice meetings. It's useful to know when your colleagues consult and visit, when you may be without a practice nurse and, for registrars, when you are without trainer support. You should know who else is doing sessions in the practice, e.g. consultants and counsellors, when they do their sessions and how to refer patients to them.

Find out the system for booking leave and swapping 'duty doctor' sessions. Let the practice manager know of any holiday or study leave you need in the near future.

PRACTICE SYSTEMS

Find out how the practice 'systems' work (*Box 4.5*). The importance of water-tight practice systems is highlighted in *Chapter 21: Guidance for good professional practice*.

Box 4.5   Practice systems

- Paperwork (see *Chapter 12*)
- Messages from patients and professionals
- Repeat prescribing (see *Chapter 8*)
- Emergency requests from patients
- Visit request protocols (see *Chapter 14*)
- What to do in an emergency
- Ordering and administration of controlled drugs (see *Chapter 8*)
- Chronic disease recall

IT TRAINING

All new members of the team should be given protected IT training. This is essential, given that much of the general practice administration, consultation and income revolve around the computer. Make sure you know your passwords, have an NHS email connection, know how to use the computer in consultations and all the other roles of the computer in primary care. You will probably need several IT training sessions over the first few weeks when you start consulting*.

See Chapter 9: Medical records and computers.

Don't worry if learning how to use the computer seems overwhelming to start with, find out who to approach when you have difficulties and appreciate that you'll learn a huge amount in the first few weeks.

SITTING IN

New team members often have the opportunity to sit in/visit with all PHCT members, and this is mandatory for all new registrars. You could also arrange visits to other community services such community pharmacist, funeral director, podiatrist, optician and social services†.

†See *Chapter 2: Working in the team.*

Whole sessions of passive observation can be quite wearing so have some objectives and prepare some questions when you sit in. Compare:

- consulting styles and speed

- the types of patients seen
- prescribing patterns
- referral patterns

Find out the special interests and responsibilities of team members.

TIME IN RECEPTION

New team members often find it useful to spend some time working in reception to experience the day to day work of the frontline staff. This is a way to appreciate not only the work of the reception team but also to familiarize you with the practice systems. Deal with phone calls, appointments, patient registrations, repeat prescribing, post, results, scanning, filing, etc.

You may also find it useful to sit in the waiting room to have some idea of the patient experience before you are known to the patients.

GP REGISTRAR'S WORKLOAD

> **GP Registrars must always be supervised whenever they are on duty**

Although as a GPR you will make a significant clinical contribution to the practice you should be always be considered as a supernumerary team member and not a workhorse! You should agree your timetable with your trainer at the start of the year but may need to renegotiate as you go along to maximise the training and educational benefits of the year.

GPRs should not be expected to:

- work more than the average full-timer at the practice, including OOH work*, *pro rata* for part-timers. Time spent on your educational commitments is considered part of your working hours

  *See *Chapter 15: Out of hours work.*

- be used as a substitute for a locum
- be involved in work that generates private income for the practice unless it is of educational value to you.

SOURCES AND FURTHER READING

1. GP Registrars guidance on BMA website, www.bma.org.uk
2. JCPTGP. *A Guide to Certification 2004*, www.jcptgp.org.uk
3. Postgraduate Medical Education and Training board, www.pmetb.org.uk
4. National Office of Summative Assessment, www.nosa.org.uk
5. Royal College of General Practitioners website, www.rcgp.org.uk

Chapter 5
Contract and finances

INTRODUCTION

This chapter covers the basic information you need about your contract and pay. More detailed advice is available from the BMA, your deanery and PCO.

GP registrars are employed by the training practice and should have an employment contract with them. The practice is reimbursed the cost of the registrar's salary*.

Qualified GPs may work in a variety of ways within a practice[†].

Before starting your post discuss your salary and contract with the practice manager if you are employed by the practice or the Human Resources department if you are employed by a PCO.

GP principals are usually self-employed and financial arrangements are covered in their practice agreement.

Use your induction period to get your basic employment administration underway[‡].

The guidance in this chapter is based on English regulations and there may be variations in other UK countries.

*Educational contracts are discussed in *Chapter 16: Educational aspects of the GP registrar year.*

†See *Chapter 1: Working in general practice* – Types of GP and *Chapter 23: Career options for general practitioners.*

‡See *Chapter 4: Starting at the practice.*

**See *Sources and further reading.*

††See *Chapter 23: Career options for general practitioners.*

CONTRACT OF EMPLOYMENT

You should be provided with a contract of employment when you start at the practice and your employer has a legal responsibility to provide one within 8 weeks of your start date (*Box 5.1*).

The BMA provides model contracts on their website for registrars, retainers, GPs working on the flexible career scheme, and other salaried GPs in GMS practices, and recommends that all salaried GPs should be employed on terms and conditions no less favourable than in their model contracts. They advise PMS practices to use the same guidance. The BMA also provides personalised advice to members through their regional offices and *askBMA***. Make sure your practice uses these model contracts as a basis for your contract.

Your contract may be amended provided you and your employers agree, though you may want to seek advice from your BMA regional office or a lawyer before doing this.

GPRs should obtain separate contracts for each GPR post they undertake if not doing a continuous 12-month stretch in the same practice, or if they are with the same practice for two or more distinct periods.

Leave

Employed doctors should usually be entitled to 25–30 working days leave in a year, *pro rata* for part-time posts, and public holidays.

If you are working as a locum you will not usually receive the benefits of paid leave and this should be reflected in the rates you charge[††].

Box 5.1   Contract of employment – key inclusions

Basic stipulations
- Job title
- Job plan to be reviewed annually
- Start date
- Notice of termination from either side, usually 3 months

Professional requirements
- Full GMC registration and licence (see *Chapter 20: Appraisal and revalidation*)
- Inclusion on PCO Medical Performers List (see *Chapter 4: Starting at the practice*)
- MPO membership

Financial
- Salary (see later), reviewed annually
- Option to contribute to NHS pension scheme (see later)

Hours
- Full time is normally 37.5 hours divided into 9 sessions, *pro rata* for part-time
- No more than 48 hours a week unless you have signed a waiver to the European Working Time Directive

Leave allowance (see later)
- Annual leave, usually 30 working days in a year, *pro rata* for part-time
- Public bank holidays
- Study leave
- Sick leave
- Maternity and paternity leave
- Parental and dependant leave
- Other leave

Health and safety
- Pre-employment medical assessment
- Agreement to abide by health and safety procedures

Additional in the GPR contract
Timetable – hours to include
- OOH (see *Chapter 15: Out of hours work*)
- Tuition
- Assessment
- VTS release course
- Minimum half day off

Box 5.1 *continued*

Duties and responsibilities
Trainer to:
- Teach and advise on all GP relevant matters
- Ensure supervision whenever GPR on duty
- Cover all message-taking service costs

Registrar to:
- Live at agreed address
- Keep and maintain suitable transport
- Keep medical records of all patient contacts
- Protect practice and patient confidentiality
- Negotiate with trainer on all other outside work activities, whether paid or not

Study leave

GPRs should have a minimum of 30 days a year of study leave. This includes the VTS release course which usually takes approximately 15 days, leaving 15 additional days. This does not include the weekly tutorial in the practice. Your contract should stipulate your total allowance which will depend on your educational needs balanced with the needs of your practice, which may take precedence. As the registrar year is an educational opportunity your trainer should look favourably on study leave applications that could further your education.

Full time salaried GPs should be offered the one session a week or equivalent for continuing professional development (CPD), *pro rata* for part-time posts.

Newly qualified GPs may be entitled to an educational allowance under 'Higher Professional Education (HPE)' schemes. These schemes are designed to encourage this group of GPs to focus on their personal training needs. They are funded by deaneries and vary around the country. You may be entitled to locum costs and course fee reimbursements for study leave. Contact your deanery for more information.

Sick leave

Sick leave allowance depends what you negotiate with the practice but should reflect your number of years of continuous NHS service. It should allow for:

- **1st year of NHS service**, 1 month full pay, 2 months half pay
- **2nd year of NHS service**, 2 months full and 2 months half pay
- **3rd year of NHS service**, 4 months full and 4 months half pay

- **4th and 5th years of NHS service**, 5 months full and 5 months half pay
- **6th and subsequent years of NHS service** 6 months full and 6 months half pay

The practice will require a self-certificate for sickness up to 7 days or a Med 3 from your GP for longer periods*.

An absence of more than 2 weeks in your registrar year will mean extending the training period accordingly.

*See *Chapter 12: Paperwork, certificates and benefits.*

Maternity leave

Maternity leave entitlement will depend on your length of service in the NHS but usually is up to 52 weeks including a period of paid leave.

The BMA model contract has clear advice on maternity leave and should be used as a minimum standard. The PCO will usually reimburse practices a locum allowance for retainers, returners, assistants and principals. Discuss maternity leave with your practice manager and seek advice from the BMA before signing your contract to maximise your paid entitlements.

The PCO will reimburse practices for GP registrars taking maternity leave to the value of 8 weeks full pay less Statutory Maternity Pay (SMP) and 14 weeks half pay.

A standard NHS maternity leave would usually include:

- 8 weeks full pay (less SMP or maternity allowance (MA))
- 14 weeks half pay (plus SMP or MA if the total does not exceed full pay)
- 4 weeks at standard SMP/MA rate

Your practice manager will need a MATB1 certificate from you from week 20†.

†See *Chapter 12: Paperwork, certificates and benefits* – Maternity certificates.

After leave, registrars are entitled to continue training with the same trainer for the remainder of the training period.

Practices should allow pregnant employees time off for antenatal care, but should be given as much notice as possible.

Locums do not usually receive maternity leave payments but you should be entitled to SMP or MA.

Paternity leave

You should be able to take up to 2 weeks paternity leave, though depending on who you work for and what's in your contract this may or may not be paid.

Parental and dependant leave

If you have worked for an employer for 12 months, you are entitled to statutory parental leave of at least 13 weeks (this is unpaid leave) for each child born or adopted after 1999. The leave must be taken in periods of not less than a week and before the child's fifth birthday.

Employees also have the right to take a few days to deal with an emergency situation involving a dependant, i.e. child, spouse or parent.

Other leave

GPs, including registrars, should be allowed paid leave to represent their colleagues on, for example, a BMA standing committee. Make sure you have discussed this with the practice team and give as much notice as possible.

Compassionate leave, paid or otherwise, needs to negotiated with your practice.

Other contractual stipulations

Transport

Your contract may require that you have your own suitable transport for visits, not necessarily a car, and that you must keep it serviced and appropriately insured. Let your insurer know that you are using it for business purposes.

A bicycle may be suitable if your practice area is not extensive but check the practice agrees.

Salaried GPs and principals should keep a mileage diary and all receipts relating to transport costs for their tax return.

Registrars should have a motor vehicle allowance included in their contract.

Medical equipment

*See *Chapter 6: Practical preparations for clinical work –* Your doctor's bag.

The practice should provide all equipment and clinical supplies for your day to day work, but may require you to buy your own medical equipment and medical bag*. These work-related costs are tax deductible expenses, so keep receipts.

Health and safety

You may be required to complete a medical assessment, usually a questionnaire, with the possibility of a medical examination prior to starting. Your employer may also request a further assessment if they become concerned about your health or fitness. Release of your medical records is only done with your signed consent.

You should be able to provide evidence of recent hepatitis B immunization status.

Breaches of contract

If your practice is in breach of your contract discuss this early with the practice manager, partners or trainer if you are a registrar (*Box 5.2*).

If you cannot resolve things in the practice, salaried doctors should seek advice from the local LMC or PCO, the BMA if they are members, or a lawyer.

Registrars could also seek advice from the VTS course organiser and/or the Deanery.

Disciplinary procedure

Very rarely a practice may have a serious performance problem with a registrar or other employed doctor, e.g. misconduct, breaching confidentiality, being under the influence of alcohol or drugs, etc., which could lead to suspension. Seek advice and support straight away from the same sources suggested in the above section if the practice initiates any type of disciplinary procedure against you.

PAY

Refer to *Chapter 4: Starting at the practice* – Personal administration, for what the practice manager will need from you before you can be paid.

Registrars

GPR salaries are agreed nationally and pay scales in England are set out in the DOH statement *Directions to Strategic Health Authorities Concerning GP Registrars* which can be found at the back of the monthly magazine *Medeconomics* which all practice managers usually get, and it can also be found on the DOH website.

Your starting salary depends on your previous NHS post and how long you have been working in the NHS. Exceptions exist where your previous post was a locum, overseas, non-consultant career grade or in public health, the private sector, or an academic post.

Your salary includes a GPR OOH supplement, calculated at a percentage of the basic salary.

Salaried GPs

The Doctors and Dentists Remuneration Body (DDRB) annually suggests a minimum range of salary for full-time salaried GPs. *Medeconomics* publishes suggested salary scales for PCO-employed GPs and *BMJ Careers* has advertised posts with salaries. Use these as guides when negotiating your pay with a practice. Take into consideration your experience, qualifications, leave allowance, length of surgeries, paperwork and visit commitment when negotiating your pay.

Allowances and reimbursements

GP registrars are entitled to a wide range of allowances and reimbursements (*Box 5.3*). You will need to provide evidence of payment, and in the case of course fees, of attendance, to your practice manager or deanery to claim these. Keep receipts and copies of the paperwork in case of non-payment.

Study leave reimbursements

Each GPR has an allocated Educational Allowance for approved courses, travel and subsistence expenses. Deanery-run courses which are already subsidised are not usually eligible for further reimbursement.

You will need to discuss and secure approval from your trainer before applying to a course. Apply for reimbursement using the deanery claim form and submit the receipt and certificate of attendance.

Box 5.3 GPR allowances and reimbursements

Allowances
- London weighting in defined zone
- Motor vehicle allowance

Reimbursements
- Medical protection organisation subscription
- Phone:
    cost of installing a bedroom phone extension (if essential for your work)
    cost of rental charge for your home phone if you pay it
- Course fees for deanery-approved courses
- Removal and associated relocation expenses for the GPR post
- Travel and subsistence for:
    searching for accommodation
    attending interview for GPR post
    sitting a postgraduate qualification (but not exam fees)
    attending an approved study leave course

Postgraduate qualification examination fees

These are not eligible for reimbursement, but you can claim for travel and subsistence costs incurred in taking the exam by applying to the Strategic Health Authority on a specific form (GPCF3).

TAX

Employees should have their tax deducted at source but you may still want to complete a tax return to maximise your tax allowances (*Box 5.4*). Remember you must declare 'additional fees', e.g. cremation forms and any medical reports which are not taxed at source.

Consider employing an accountant with an interest in general practice. General advice is available on the BMA website.

Self-employed GPs will need to keep aside some of their income for paying tax. You will have to complete a tax return and may find an accountant's input essential. You are able to claim back all travel costs, courses, books, use of your home for work purposes and other work-related expenses against your tax. Keep all receipts and payment details.

Salaried doctors may have these costs paid in full by their employer, otherwise include them on your tax return as they may be tax deductible*.

*See *Chapter 23: Career options for general practitioners.*

Box 5.4   General tax-allowable medical expenses

Consult your accountant for your personal tax position

Professional fees
- GMC annual retention fee
- BMA membership
- Annual membership fees of Royal Colleges
- Medical indemnity

Medical equipment
Computers
Work related travel costs
Work related phone costs

Some of these costs may be payable by your employer if you are salaried.

NATIONAL INSURANCE

Employed GPs should have NI deducted from salary at source. Check this on your first payslip.

*See *Chapter 23: Career options for general practitioners –* Locums, Money matters.

Self-employed locums and principals should get in touch with the Inland Revenue NI Contributions Office to arrange payment of their regular NI payments*.

PENSIONS

The NHS superannuation scheme is recognised as a good scheme into which most NHS doctors pay. Your pay slips should include details of pension deductions.

As a registrar, salaried GP or GP principal you can choose to pay into the NHS scheme and you should organize this with your practice manager

GP locum work is now eligible for inclusion in the NHS scheme, though there have been complaints that the benefits are not as good as for GP principals. GP locums must be on the performers list and apply to the PCO or SHA to make pension contributions. Ninety per cent of gross locum income is pensionable, 10% is considered costs for professional expenses. Work must be in the NHS, not through a third party such as an agency and you must keep and be prepared to submit exact details of what work you did, when, for whom and how much you were paid.

All doctors contributing to the NHS superannuation scheme should receive an annual statement, SD86, from the NHS Pension Agency. Contact them if you have any queries about your pension or payments.

SOURCES AND FURTHER READING

1. British Medical Association, www.bma.org.uk
2. askBMA@bma.org.uk, telephone 0870 6060828.
3. Department of Health, www.dh.gov.uk
4. Department of Health, *Directions to Strategic Health Authorities concerning GP Registrars*, November 2003.
5. The Review Body Doctor and Dentists Remuneration at the Office of Manpower Economics, www.ome.uk.com
6. *Medeconomics* journal, www.medeconomics.co.uk
7. *British Medical Journal Careers*, www.bmjcareers.com
8. NHS Pensions Agency, www.nhspa.gov.uk
9. National Association of Sessional GPs, www.nasgp.org.uk
10. Inland Revenue National Contributions Agency, www.inlandrevenue.gov.uk
11. Locum Doctor Survival Pack available at www.locum123.com

Chapter 6
Practical preparations for clinical work

INTRODUCTION

Use your induction period to sort out your consulting room, medical bag and start collecting your reference material. This chapter makes recommendations on what you are likely to need and is based on our personal experience and the drugs and equipment provided at our local OOH centre.

New GPs will need to buy a medical bag and some diagnostic equipment, the practice should provide clinical supplies and paperwork. Borrow equipment from the practice before you buy anything. Check out the medical supplies catalogues and equipment mail order section at the back of the GP newspapers which may be cheaper than specialist medical shops. Keep all your receipts for tax purposes.

Some OOH services provide all equipment and drugs for use in their sessions.

YOUR BAG

Your doctor's bag must be lockable and not too heavy. Anything advertised as a medical bag may be expensive and offer no advantages over a cheaper alternative such as a briefcase, toolbox, or vanity case.

If you have to leave it in your car make sure both the bag, and the car, are locked.

> **You are responsible for your own bag so re-stock it regularly**

Equipment and clinical supplies

Unless you have a double set of everything, your main equipment will be used both in surgery and on daytime visits. How much you carry will (*Box 6.1*) depend in part on where you practice. GPs working in remote areas may need more emergency equipment than inner-city GPs working close to A&E.

Drugs for your bag

> **Regularly check drugs are in date**

There is an essential minimum you must carry for potentially life-threatening conditions such as MI, cardiac arrest, asthma, anaphylaxis, hypoglycaemia or meningococcal infection. Our suggestions (see *Boxes 6.2 and 6.3*) here are based on *The Drug and Therapeutics Bulletin's* 'Drugs for the doctor's bag (2000)' and 'Parenteral Doses of Drugs for Medical Emergencies'.

Box 6.1   Supplies for your medical bag

Equipment
- Stethoscope
- Portable sphygmomanometer
- Ophthalmoscope/auriscope and pen torch
- Thermometer
- Spacer, peak flow meter, mouthpieces and PEFR calculator
- Patella hammer
- Tape measure
- Laerdal pocket mask and oropharyngeal airway
- Scissors

Clinical supplies
- Drugs (see *Boxes 6.2 and 6.3*)
- Empty medicine bottles (or envelopes)
- Tongue depressors
- Microbiology swabs
- Urine specimen pots
- Urinalysis sticks
- Paediatric urine sampling bags
- Gloves including a sterile pair, lubricating jelly, tissues
- Lancets and glucometer
- Venesection/injection equipment
- i.v. cannulae
- Disinfecting swabs
- Pregnancy test kit and gestation calculator
- Dressing pack and some simple dressings and tape
- Fluorescein strips
- Specimen bags

General
- Sharps box
- Rubbish receptacle
- Disinfecting wet wipes

Paperwork
- Prescription pad, headed notepaper, envelopes, pathology and radiology forms, Mental Health Section papers
- List of practice and hospital phone numbers (see inside back cover)
- X-ray and pathology request forms
- Emergency drug dose list
- Notebook

Books
- *BNF*
- Local map

For remoter areas
- Nebuliser and defibrillator
- i.v. cannulae, fluids and giving set
- Suture pack
- Speculum
- Fetal stethoscope/doppler

*See *Chapter 8: Prescribing –*
Controlled drugs.

Update yourself with the regulations on the carriage and storage of controlled drugs (CDs)*. Doctors have been prosecuted for contravening these regulations so you *must* observe them.

Ordering drug supplies

Your drugs may come from practice stocks or be ordered from the pharmacist. This may be the role of one of the nurses or administrative staff, otherwise you will need to liaise with the pharmacist directly. Drugs for stock and bags are ordered on a private prescription† and charged to the practice or individual doctor.

†See *Chapter 8: Prescribing –*
Private prescription.

Try to keep limited supplies of drugs. You rarely use them and they go out of date. Most patients will have access to a pharmacy within 24–48 hours of a visit.

Dispensing drugs from your bag

Transfer drugs from your supplies into spare medicine bottles or an envelope. Label the container clearly with the patient's name, date, full drug and dose details and the number of tablets supplied. Remind the patient to store drugs safely.

Document in the medical records the batch number, expiry date and, if appropriate, manufacturer of any drugs you actually administer yourself, particularly injections or vaccinations‡.

‡See *Chapter 8: Prescribing –*
Drug and product liability.

Other preparations for visiting

You are required to have a car or other suitable transport and a mobile phone is essential. Street parking regulations for doctors vary so check with your practice manager for local arrangements. Have little to identify your vehicle as a doctor's to reduce break-ins.

For personal safety consider carrying a personal alarm and carry very limited supplies of drugs and prescriptions, though bear in mind attacks on GPs are not common.

YOUR CONSULTING ROOM

Ideally you should have your own consulting room, which should be cleared of your predecessor's paraphernalia and re-stocked for your arrival (*Box 6.4*). If you have to share a room, or move between rooms, devise a system to keep your personal affairs and paperwork separate and clearly identifiable as yours, a trolley or plastic basket should do.

Make your room comfortable and safe both for you and your patients. All sharps bins and dangerous equipment should be out of children's reach and prescriptions and medical certificate pads should be kept out of sight.

Box 6.2   Emergency drugs

Remember vials of water for injection

Condition	Drug (refer to *BNF* for doses)
Anaphylaxis	Epinephrine (Adrenaline) 1 ml (1 in 1000) Chlorpheniramine 1 ml (10 mg/ml) injection Hydrocortisone powder (as succinate) 100 mg Also for asthma and hypoadrenalism
Asthma (carry a spacer device)	Salbutamol nebules 2.5 ml (1 mg/ml) *or* Terbutaline nebules 2 ml (2.5 mg/ml) Salbutamol or terbutaline inhaler Prednisolone 5 mg soluble tablets Hydrocortisone powder (as succinate) 100 mg
Cardiac: Suspected MI	Aspirin 300 mg tablets (soluble or chewable) GTN spray Diamorphine 5 mg Metoclopramide 2 ml (5 mg/ml) or Cyclizine 1 ml (50 mg/ml)
Acute LVF	Furosemide 5 ml (10 mg/ml) Diamorphine
Bradycardia	Atropine 1 ml (600 µg/ml)
Diabetic hypoglycaemia	Glucose tablets or 3 sugar lumps (= 10 g) or Hypostop gel Glucagon 1 mg/ml injection Glucose i.v. solution 50 ml of 20%
Epileptic fit or Febrile convulsion (also useful for psychotic agitation)	Rectal diazepam 1.25 ml (2 mg/ml) and Rectal diazepam 2.5 ml (2 mg/ml) *or* Diazepam emulsion 2 ml (5 mg/ml) vial × 1
Meningococcal disease	Benzylpenicillin 2 × 600 mg ('GP Pack') For confirmed penicillin allergy: Cefotaxime 1g vial or Chloramphenicol 1g vial
Psychiatric: agitated psychotic	Chlorpromazine 1 ml (25 mg/ml) vial or Haloperidol 1 ml (5 mg/ml) vial (can also be used for vomiting)
Antidotes	Flumazenil 5 ml (100 µg/ml) vial Naloxone 1 ml (400 µg/ml) vial Procyclidine 2 ml (5 mg/ml) vial
Analgesia	Diamorphine as above Tramadol 2 ml (50 mg/ml) Diclofenac 3 ml (25 mg/ml) vial

"Drugs for the Doctor's Bag Revisited" – *Drug and Therapeutics Bulletin*, (Vol. 38, No. 9, September 2000) reproduced with kind permission from Consumers' Association, 2 Marylebone Rd, London, NW1 4DF.

Find out if a staff member is responsible for re-stocking your room or if you are expected to do this yourself.

Your desktop

A cluttered desk can easily add to your sense of chaos so try to keep your desktop and drawers organised. Although more forms are available electronically a lot of paper is still necessary* (*Box 6.5*). Devise a system to process your incoming and outgoing paperwork and for items pending. Keep to hand a notebook/electronic organiser for your to-do list, patient queries and results to follow up.

Find out about any practice policy on shredding and recycling.

*See *Chapter 12: Paperwork, certificates and benefits.*

Box 6.4   Clinical equipment for the consulting room

As for your medical bag (*Box 6.1*) plus:

Equipment
- Weighing scales
- Height meter
- Snellen chart with correct distance marked

Clinical supplies
- Disposable and sterile gloves
- Stool specimen pots
- Microbiology, chlamydia, virology swabs
- Gynaecology examination: specula, spatulae, cytobrush, slides, fixative, pencil, slide carriers
- Tuning fork
- Monofilament for diabetic foot checks
- Sharps bin

Box 6.5   Stationery

- Headed notepaper, envelopes and compliments slips
- Prescriptions
- Pathology, radiology, cardiology request forms
- Medical certificates
- Printer paper
- Referral forms for local services
- Prescription charge exemption application forms
- Termination of pregnancy form HSA1
- Practice leaflets

Access to:
- Death certificates and cremation forms
- Mental health section papers
- Notifiable disease certificate book
- Vaccination summary cards

(See also *Boxes 12.4 and 12.6 in Chapter 12: Paperwork, certificates and benefits*)

REFERENCE MATERIAL

Box 6.6 is a suggested list for clinical reference material, some of which may be available electronically. Use the telephone number list suggested inside the back cover and the websites in Appendix 1.

Box 6.6   Clinical reference materials (+/– on computer)

Clinical
- Pregnancy gestation calculator
- Peak flow prediction calculator
- BMI calculator
- Children's growth charts
- Travel vaccinations/malaria prophylaxis charts
- Local prescribing guidelines
- Practice protocols
- CVD risk calculator

Administrative
- Internal phone extensions
- Local hospitals directory
- List of private consultants/hospitals

Publications
- The *BNF* or *MIMS*
- *Clinical Evidence*
- Clinical guidelines
- NICE guidelines summary
- Practice or local formulary if available
- Guide to 'Over the Counter' (OTC) drugs
- *Department of Health Immunisation Against Infectious Disease* –'The Green book'
- *Department of Health Guide to Travel Vaccinations* –'The Yellow book'
- Fitness to Drive *'At A Glance'* guide

SOURCES AND FURTHER READING

1. Drugs for the Doctor's Bag Revisited including insert 'Parenteral Doses of Drugs for Medical Emergencies', *Drug and Therapeutic Bulletin*, **38**: 2000.
2. Current *British National Formulary*, www.bnf.org
3. *Clinical Evidence*, BMJ Publishing, www.clinicalevidence.com

4. NICE guidelines summary, www.nice.org.uk
5. Practice or local formulary.
6. Proprietary Association of Great Britain *Guide to 'Over the Counter' (OTC) Drugs.*
7. Department of Health. *Health Information for Overseas Travellers.* HMSO 2001 ('The Yellow Book').
8. Department of Health. *Immunisation Against Infectious Disease.* HMSO 1996 ('The Green Book').
9. Fitness to Drive *'At A Glance'* guide, available at www.dvla.gov.uk
10. Drug Tariff, available on Prescription Pricing Authority website, www.ppa.org.uk

Chapter 7
The consultation: survival tips for the new GP

INTRODUCTION

There is no right or wrong way to consult, nor is there a perfect consultation. You will develop your own individual style with experience and this will evolve throughout your working life.

This chapter highlights some of the issues we found problematic when we started consulting. Your own experience, input from your trainer or mentor, and reviews of videos of your consultations will fill in some of the gaps. Read the classic consultation texts (see *Sources and further reading*), though you may find them a little overwhelming at the outset. When you can run your surgeries safely and comfortably use these texts to refine your technique. Start with a simple guide to communication skills.

Management of specific clinical problems are well-covered elsewhere and are not covered here.

STARTING OFF

Fundamental features of general practice consultations are:

- seeing pathology at an early, often unclear stage, and developing over time
- distinguishing the serious problems from the less serious
- dealing with uncertainty

The transition to GP consulting

Presentations in general practice are often less well defined than in secondary care so a different approach is needed. The main difference between hospital and general practice consultations are:

- Full clerkings are rarely required. The medical record should already hold a summary of the medical history. Most new GPs try to hang on to hospital type clerkings initially and are given longer consulting time partly to account for this.
- Relatively few presentations lend themselves to a clear diagnosis.
- Patients often present with several problems at once.
- Most presentations do not need sorting out immediately (aside from the few medical emergencies) despite anxiety generated by worried patients. You rarely need to rush out on a visit and you should resist being pressured into prompt action by socially inconvenienced patients.
- Test results, and patients, take time to come back. There is no consultant ward round to gear up for (you are now the consultant!) and so there is always the potential to lose patients to follow up. Learn to share responsibility with patients for follow up of their medical problems and results. You cannot keep track of every patient in the way you are expected to as a house officer but you should keep a record of those you need to be sure have been followed up.

- Every consultation doesn't need to end with a prescription, investigation or referral. Simple reassurance and masterly inactivity may be often be the best option but may feel rather unsettling at first.
- Always remember 'There are some patients you cannot help, there are no patients you cannot harm'*.

*See Sources and further reading.

Your early surgeries and getting up to speed

Your first solo surgeries should be very light to allow for the fact you are still in hospital clerking mode and unfamiliar with the patient, computer and general practice medicine. You should progress to shorter appointment times as your confidence increases. Registrars should be able to manage a surgery load similar to that of their trainer including added urgent cases by the end of the registrar year. Work up to this by about month four to six but resist pressure to do so until you are ready.

You will run late: almost all GPs do and you will get quicker with experience. People are naturally fast or slow consulters and trying to change from one type to the other is likely to induce a lot of stress and may be counterproductive. However, if running late is a persistent problem then registrars should discuss it with their trainer. You may need to make some adjustments to your approach, what you are trying to achieve in the consultation and how you organise yourself.

New GPs should not be surprised if they feel totally exhausted in their first few weeks although often working fewer hours than in hospital jobs. This can be the result of unfamiliar clinical material, intense patient contact and the emotionally draining content of some consultations. GPs also work in relative isolation and have greater individual clinical responsibility than hospital training grade doctors. However, if you were previously a medical specialist registrar you may find it all a breeze compared to outpatients!

Your case mix

Many of the cases you see will be one-off, straightforward acute medical problems but you will acquire some regulars. Trainers should review their registrar's case mix from time to time to ensure a representative selection including patients with long term illness, ongoing psychosocial problems and someone requiring terminal care.

THE CONSULTATION ITSELF

The practical components of the consultation; completing the medical record, prescribing, certificates, investigations and referrals are dealt with individually in subsequent chapters.

Conducting the consultation

*See Chapter 6: Practical preparations for clinical work.

Your room should comfortable for you and your patients*. Glance through the medical record before calling in your patient, even if you know them well, to ensure you have the correct records to hand. Most GPs personally call patients in from the waiting room. A buzzer system is quicker but less personal.

Start the consultation with a non-directive opener such as 'What can I do for you?' Don't assume you know the reason for their attendance even if you invited the patient back for review as they may have other issues to discuss.

Give the patient uninterrupted time to tell you their reason/s for coming. Start to explore their presenting complaint by asking direct questions after a few minutes.

Try to maintain eye contact and avoid excessive bonding with the computer, notes or the clock.

If it is transpires that there are several problems ask the patient to prioritise them and make it clear you will limit the consultation to what can be covered reasonably in the time available. Limit patients to urgent problems only in an urgent appointment and invite them back for a further appointment, particularly if a detailed examination or a procedure is required.

When an examination is necessary ask the patient to undress only as much as is needed. Ideally you should offer a chaperone for all intimate examinations, even if you are the same gender.

Terminating the consultation can be an art in itself. You may sometimes need to fall back on the psychotherapist's favourite phrase: 'I'm afraid that is all we have time for today' and even walk them to the door. Most patients are very sensitive to the time limits of GPs.

Follow up and 'safety netting'

New GPs particularly will ask patients they see to come back for follow up. This is partly for review following investigations or new medication but also to reassure yourself that you are not missing something. It's also a good way to observe the natural history of many self-limiting conditions.

If you are not arranging a follow up appointment then give your patient clear advice to come back if their symptoms change or deteriorate. Advice must be specific: 'come back if the fever is not settling within three days' or 'if the breathing worsens so that the baby cannot feed easily' and document the advice given. You may sometimes agree on a time for a telephone review rather than a face to face consultation.

Some patients will inevitably leave you feeling anxious or uncertain about your management. New GPs should discuss these cases with their trainer or other partner. You can always phone a patient later to check on progress, or inform them of a revised management plan after discussion with another GP.

If you sense you will be left with some anxiety about a patient, particularly those with acute presentations, then trust your gut instinct and arrange prompt review or refer them.

As you progress as a GP aim to bring fewer patients back for follow up to free up appointments for new problems.

Only through the experience of many patient contacts can you begin to achieve a balance between:

- you own learning needs in seeing the resolution or progression of conditions, and
- handing back responsibility to the patient to return appropriately

THE CLINICAL CONTENT OF THE CONSULTATION

New GPs should be well equipped from their hospital experience to deal with presentations with a clear history and obvious pathology that require referral. Though deciding the priority of the referral and the extent to which you should investigate in general practice may present a dilemma for the newcomer. If you are unsure how to manage a presentation it is fine to look things up in front of patients; do this with confidence. Clinical decision support software can be helpful mid-consultation but you will need to spend some time familiarising yourself with how to use it.

Mid-surgery you can always ask your trainer or other doctor and afterwards you can liaise with your hospital and pharmacy colleagues as needed. Let the patient know you will contact them and don't forget to.

General practice presentations fall broadly into the following five categories.

'Bread and butter' medicine

While this includes some relatively straightforward problems, e.g. UTIs and contraception, other conditions, e.g. nappy rash and joint pains, are likely to cause problems for the new GP. They are rarely dealt with in hospitals, and generally ignored at medical school, so you will be on a steep learning curve initially. The *BNF* in particular and books on clinical general practice are very useful here together with experience, tutorials, home reading and MCQ practice.

Psychosocial problems

These crop up frequently in surgeries either overtly, e.g. as requests for housing letters or referrals for counselling, or covertly as medically unexplained symptoms. Even in cases you believe are entirely psychological you should be able to exclude a physical cause to reassure the patient and yourself.

The impact of social circumstances and mental health on general health will be a recurring theme in surgeries throughout your career.

Registrars should arrange a tutorial on the recognition and management of depression in all its guises as you will see a lot of it.

With experience you will develop skills in:

- picking up the hidden agenda, e.g. repeated attendance for 'minor problems' that may reflect an underlying problem e.g. depression
- recognising and managing psychosomatic problems
- illness associated with secondary gain, i.e. benefits of the sick role which unconsciously keeps people ill
- addressing your own personal boundaries, limitations and prejudices

Long term illness/chronic disease

GPs manage a number of long term illnesses either alone or shared with a hospital specialist. Some practices organise specific clinics for asthma, diabetes and coronary heart disease, which allow for continuity of care for the patient while reducing some of the burden on secondary care. Clinics are often run by practice nurses with GP support using practice protocols based on national or local evidence-based guidelines. Make sure you have an opportunity to participate in any such clinics. Familiarise yourself with the computer templates and prompts used*.

*See *Chapter 9: Medical records and computers* – Data entry.

Acquire a few patients with chronic diseases for follow up as they provide an ideal opportunity to develop an ongoing relationship while monitoring clinical progress.

Review the patient's medical record to be sure all new contract QOF criteria are met, and opportunistically include items in the consultation when they are not[†].

†See *Chapter 1: Working in general practice.*

Health promotion

Although this forms a large part of the practice nurse remit you should also make use of every opportunity in routine surgeries to discuss the big 'five':

- smoking
- alcohol
- diet
- exercise
- sexual health

Check and document BP, BMI, contraception, sexual health promotion, smear and vaccination due dates. Use patient information leaflets (PILs) to reinforce your advice. Always document any advice and leaflets you give.

Emergencies in general practice

Medical emergencies are much less common in the community than in hospitals, so you risk losing your skills. Make notes of your well-learned hospital management skills while they are still fresh in your mind.

The surgery drug cupboard should be well stocked to cover basic emergencies.

You may have to deal with emergencies alone, in the surgery or on a visit, without the luxury of a helpful nurse. You may also have to contend with an interested lay audience so it is useful to develop a systematic approach (*Box 7.1*).

Box 7.1   An approach to dealing with medical emergencies in general practice

- Don't panic!
- Assume control of the situation
- Summon help
- Make sure someone calls for an ambulance
- Delegate where possible
- Take time to assess the clinical situation fully
- Institute appropriate management, which may involve anything from CPR to doing nothing until an ambulance arrives
- Always wait with the patient if an ambulance is needed or ensure they are not left alone until fully recovered
- Take time to inform relatives
- Document the incident fully in the medical record
- Debrief with your trainer or other doctor
- Discuss the case at practice 'critical incident' meetings if appropriate

---

What to do when you don't know what to do

Vague presentations that don't fit a clear clinical picture, e.g. tired all the time, pain all over, are common in general practice. Sometimes it can be illuminating simply to ask the patient empathetically what they are worried about, or what help they want from you: 'what is it you were hoping I can do?' An alternative approach is to buy some time by organising some limited simple investigations, e.g. FBC, ESR/CRP, urinanalysis, and arrange a review with these results. Normal tests may well be reassuring for both you and the patient and a second consultation may also allow a hidden agenda to surface. Don't hesitate to seek advice from your colleagues.

DIFFICULT CONSULTATIONS

Not all consultations go smoothly and there may be days when you are not on top form and have a run of difficult consultations. Don't worry, it happens to us all.

Occasionally you will feel pressurised into management that you are not comfortable with, such as issuing prescriptions for benzodiazepines, or referring when you deem it unnecessary. If you feel a request from a patient is inappropriate then explain why; evidence-based medicine can help here, and 'it is our practice policy' can also be a good get-out clause provided it really is that. Try to come to a mutually agreed compromise. Open discussion may bring up other issues and help avoid a confrontation. You may need to refer the patient back to their usual GP if you feel you cannot, or do not want to, manage the request yet they are insistent. There will be times when you have to give in so don't see this as a failing and document it in the notes as 'patient insisted' to forewarn future consulters.

Breaking bad news

It is normal to dread situations where you need to communicate an abnormal result with potentially serious consequences and you may well be tempted to put it off. Here are a few tips to help.

- Prepare yourself by checking the clinical facts further, discussing the situation with your colleagues and arranging a standby management plan before seeing the patient.
- Invite the patient in for a review. Ask a member of the reception staff to phone and give them a prompt appointment or write a non-alarmist letter. Don't be surprised if they phone you in a panic on receipt of the letter. By all means have some discussion over the phone but face-to-face contact is better if there is potentially bad news. Allow plenty of time.
- Your patient may well suspect something is amiss already so probe by asking them some open questions about the situation: 'had you any thoughts about the tests and what they might show?'. Give them plenty of time to air their thoughts or fears during which they may well arrive at the bad news themselves.
- Explain the implications of the abnormal result and how reliable the test is.
- Be honest, but not brutally so and expect that they will not be able to take in much of what you say. You may need to back up your discussion with leaflets or put salient points such as the diagnosis, in writing.
- Patients may also go into denial, and you will have to find a balance between destroying this protective mechanism without colluding with them that nothing is wrong.
- Explain the management options, including any you have set up already and ask them how they wish to go from here. They may well not be in a situation to answer immediately so don't force the point now.
- Ask them how they feel about the situation, any specific fears they harbour and ask how you might be able to help allay these. Ensure they will have some support when they leave the surgery.
- Make yourself available for further discussion and book them another appointment yourself shortly afterwards to allow discussion of the

questions that inevitably arise. Suggest that they have someone accompany them when they come again.

Angry patients

Angry patients can often provoke strong feelings in you. If you find you are getting angry with a patient remember that it may be originating from them and transferring to you; try not to let this happen.

There may be understandable reasons for their anger such as illness, being kept waiting, or general distrust of medics based on previous experience, so it is worth trying to stand back to find out the underlying cause.

Reflecting back to the patient calmly that you sense they are angry may allow them to express themselves more constructively. Try phrases like 'you seem very angry about this. How were you hoping I could help?'. Acknowledging their discomfort, frustration or disappointment may also help. You will get better with experience.

Defusing a potentially violent situation

Violent situations in general practice are very unusual.

Put your safety first if you feel physically threatened and summon help using the panic button or by leaving the room. Don't worry if valuables are exposed. Get someone to call the police if the situation is escalating, or there has been violence or an assault.

If you sense a situation is getting out of hand aim to defuse it by maintaining a calm exterior and tone of voice, however scared you feel. Avoid rising to the patient's heightened state, particularly if you are being provoked by cries such as 'call yourself a bloody doctor?'.

If an error has been made then don't be too pompous to apologise. Acknowledging you may have been in the wrong can help avert a complaint and allows patients to see that you are human too, both in your error and in your ability to apologise: 'you sound very upset about ... I am sorry if ...'*.

See Chapter 21: Guidance for good professional practice.

If you really can't negotiate with the patient then state clearly: 'I can hear what you are saying but I cannot help you if you continue to behave like this' and make it clear that you are 'not happy to continue the consultation in this manner'.

Debriefing after a difficult consultation

After a particularly difficult consultation take some time out before seeing your next patient otherwise they will get short shrift. Consider going to the toilet or putting the kettle on even if you are running late. Discuss the situation fully with your colleagues after surgery and try to see it as a learning experience. Identify how else you might have handled the situation. You may find the patient has the same effect on everyone and simply has unreasonable expectations that need to be addressed by the practice as a whole.

If there has been any actual or threatened violence, document the event meticulously in the medical records. Ensure the patient's notes are flagged, relevant practice staff are informed, and consider arrangements for future consultations in secure settings if necessary. The practice may decide to remove the patient from the list. Whether or not to report the event to the police, or even press charges may be a consideration, and you should discuss this with the partners.

DIFFICULT PATIENT TYPES

Though very few patients are 'difficult' they cause a disproportionate amount of angst for GPs. It is important to put these into perspective and not let one difficult patient cast a negative shadow over all the others you see that day.

Some patients will like you and some won't no matter how hard you try. We simply cannot please all of our patients all of the time. Don't be misled by the 'flatterers', who may want special attention from you, or conversely, the 'rejectors' who don't come back and see you. These actions may be conscious or unconscious on the part of the patient.

Some patients shop-around and see every new doctor in the hope of finding the one who finally understands them. Although you might be just that doctor you are more likely to be flavour of the month then rejected like all the rest. Looking through the notes may confirm this pattern. Some patients don't mind who they see so long as they don't have to wait long.

There are some well-recognised categories of patients who present management challenges for the GP, often with lengthy and frequent consultations. Many have deep psychological difficulties which they are unable to address or even recognise, despite reflection from an astute doctor.

Heartsinks

These patients literally make your heart sink at the prospect of a consultation with them. They include four stereotypes (*Box 9.2*).

Box 9.2   Types of heartsink patients (Groves, 1978)

- Dependent clingers
- Entitled demanders
- Manipulative help-rejectors
- Self-destructive deniers.

They can produce feelings of exasperation, depression and helplessness in the doctor, which may be transference of how they themselves feel. Interestingly, patients who are heartsinks for one GP do not necessarily produce the same reaction in another doctor.

Being clear about what you can and can't provide for them may be helpful.

Somatisers

Such patients experience and complain of physical symptoms which are medically inexplicable, and usually reflect underlying distress which the patient cannot accept as an explanation.

They often have thick notes, wide-ranging and repeated specialist referrals and investigations with no substantial 'medical' problem found. They may also demand small-print investigations or to try all new or complementary treatments.

Management tips include:

- recognising the pattern
- acknowledging fully the physical symptoms and the distress they cause
- encouraging them to see the same overseeing doctor who should limit referrals

Frequent attenders

These, by definition, consult more times than the average of 3.5 consultations per patient a year. They are a very mixed group encompassing somatisers and heartsinks as well as those with multiple complex problems and physical disease. Management tips include:

- making clear problem lists
- planning regular follow up
- encouraging the patient to share responsibility for managing their health problems
- encouraging them to stick to one doctor

Manipulative patients

Some patients, particularly substance misusers, know how to 'play the system' and can be very manipulative. They may respond to firm boundaries such as a mutual contract setting out the circumstances under which they will and will not be treated. This can help them to share some responsibility for their actions. If they don't stick to the contract, they won't get what they want so don't give in! You will develop the experience and confidence to do this as your career progresses.

Don't be put off by threats: it is *not* your fault if patients use street drugs because you wouldn't give them valium or whatever else they demand. Sympathise with their distress but remind them they have choices over their actions. Offer to make arrangements for longer term plans such as arranging rehabilitation.

We all get pressurised into agreeing prescriptions from time to time so give only short courses for a few days if you can't avoid prescribing.

GIFTS FROM PATIENTS

Though it may be gratifying to receive gifts and thank you letters from grateful patients it is not without its problems. Be wary of the occasional patient who regularly showers you with gifts in the hope of gaining special attention. If you suspect this is the case then address it sensitively otherwise it may hamper effective doctor–patient communication.

Your practice should have a policy on gifts. Under the nGMS, the practice must keep a register of any gift over £100, and it may be wise to include less valuable gifts especially if an individual gives small repeated gifts. Gifts include hospitality from drug companies.

If a patient does want to give a gift, suggest they buy something for the benefit of the practice or make a donation to charity; advise them that all gifts have to be included in the register.

Some practices will divide all the chocolates and alcohol received at Christmas amongst all the practice staff.

It is a good idea to keep a personal file or record of any gifts or letters you receive. Look through them on bad days to remind yourself of patients' appreciation.

PERSONAL QUESTIONS FROM PATIENTS

GPs vary as to how much personal information they are prepared to divulge to their patients. Enquiries about your age, residence and whether you can be called by your first name are not uncommon and can be awkward to deal with. A helpful phrase can be 'we're here to talk about you today' to divert overly personal questions. Though many GPs are friends with some of their patients, remember that it can be difficult to treat them as objectively as you would your other patients and they may expect special favours from you.

SOURCES AND FURTHER READING

1. Risdale L. *Evidence-based General Practice, A Critical Reader*. Saunders, 1996.
2. Neighbour R. *The Inner Consultation*. Kluwer Academic Publishers, 1987.
3. Tate P. *The Doctor's Communication Handbook,* 4th Edition. Radcliffe Medical Press, 2002.
4. Pendleton D. *et al. The New Consultation,* 2nd Edition. Oxford University Press, 2003.

5. Balint M. *The Doctor, His Patient and the Illness*, 3rd Edition. Churchill Livingstone, 2000.
6. Rosenthal J. *et al. The Successful GP Registrar's Companion.* Churchill Livingstone, 2003.
7. Groves J.E. Taking care of the hateful patient. *New Engl. J. Med.* **298**: 883–887, 1978.
8. Gill D., Sharpe M. Frequent Consulters in General Practice: a systematic review of studies of prevalence, associations and outcome. *J. Psychosom. Res.* **47**: 115–130.
9. Helman C. *Culture Health and Illness: An Introduction for Health Professionals.* Hodder Arnold, 2000.
10. Coales U. Dealing with 'heartsink' patients. *BMJ Careers Focus* **329**: 203, 2004.
11. Cuervo L.G., Aronson J.K. The road to healthcare. *BMJ* **329**: 1–2, 2004.

Chapter 8
Prescribing

INTRODUCTION

> **You have legal and clinical responsibility for any prescription you sign. Do not sign any you are not entirely confident about, particularly if they are initiated or generated by someone else**

Prescribing in primary care is a hugely expensive and complex area of health provision. In 2003 650 million items were prescribed costing over £7 billion and accounting for 14% of the entire NHS budget.

Each consultation need not end with a prescription ('script') but many do. In 1998, 69% of patients consulting a GP received a prescription. A recommendation for an OTC preparation may be more appropriate and can save money both for patients who pay for their prescriptions and the NHS.

As a new GP you will need to concentrate on matching appropriate medication to condition but your awareness of prescribing protocols, generic prescribing and drug costs should increase as you progress.

The nGMS contract promotes safe medicines management by allocating a number of quality points to the medication review and safe prescribing systems in the practice*.

*See *Chapter 1: Working in general practice.*
Further prescribing tips are given in:
Chapter 6: Practical preparations for clinical work – Your bag.
Chapter 9: Medical records and computers – Prescribing on the computer.
Chapter 15: Out of hours work – Using drugs out of hours.

GOOD PRESCRIBING PRACTICE

You must always aim to adhere to good prescribing practice (*Box 8.2*). Medication errors account for a large number of hospital admissions, complaints, and medico-legal claims. Try to be sure your patient understands what they are being prescribed, what side effects to look out for and what adverse effects to report. It is useful to give patients a list of their current medication.

Box 8.1   Common prescribing mistakes

- wrong dosage
- right drug prescribed to the wrong patient
- inappropriate repeat prescribing (see later)
- new drug interacts with existing medication
- inappropriate medication
- failure to monitor treatment
- failure of communication between doctor and patient
- an item is prescribed but not required

Box 8.2   Good prescribing practice

- Consider carefully whether the treatment is really indicated
- Always carry and consult with a current *BNF*
- Prescribe safely, so check specifically for:
  - known allergies
  - interactions and polypharmacy
  - pregnancy and breast feeding
- Prescribe generically unless medically inappropriate (see below)
- Avoid combination formulations (except oral contraception and HRT)
- Abide by existing practice formularies or prescribing protocols
- Be aware of maximum duration of treatment per prescription
- Limit the amount of drug you issue for known drug misusers or where you doubt the genuineness of request
- Document all treatment fully in the medical record with review arrangements
- Document medication reviews
- Update prescribing records following home visits, OOH contacts and specialist reviews
- Develop an awareness of drug costs (but remember cheaper is *not* always better)

Aim for evidence-based, cost-effective and safe prescribing with a fully counselled patient. Keep up with the latest evidence-based guidelines, use drug information sources (see *Sources and further reading*) and develop a good relationship with your community pharmacist and PCO prescribing team.

WRITING PRESCRIPTIONS

GP prescriptions are made on the FP10 form or its computer equivalent FP10Comp. These are issued by the Prescription Pricing Authority and bear the GP principal's name, prescribing number, surgery address and telephone number so all prescriptions can be traced.

Named GPs, including all principals, have a prescribing number and should sign their own allocated prescriptions whereas registrars and some non-principals prescribe under their trainer's or another principal's name, but still maintain responsibility for each script they sign. If your name is not on the FP10 add it in block capitals to your signature so the pharmacist can identify you as the prescriber should any queries arise.

Box 8.3　Accurate completion of prescriptions

- Use indelible ink
- Patient's full name and address, plus age (essential if 12 years or under) or date of birth
- Medicine name
- Medicine formulation (tablet, capsule, soluble, syrup, suppository, cream, patch)
- Route (p.o., p.r., p.v., sublingual, buccal, topical, transdermal)
- Dose – write out micrograms or nanograms in full, avoid the use of decimals and when used always ensure a 0 goes before the dot i.e. 0.5 ml not .5 ml)
- Frequency
- Total quantity or duration of course
- Your signature (and print your name if not your prescription)
- Date

o.d. = once daily
b.d. = twice
t.d.s. = three times
q.d.s. = four times
p.r.n. = as required (pharmacists prefer specific instructions)
o.p. = standard pack size or tube of cream

Accurate completion of prescriptions is detailed above (*Box 8.3*). Your computer prescribing programme will also give you helpful prompts. Familiarise yourself with the information on the reverse of the FP10 as you may occasionally need to complete this on behalf of your patients.

Prescriptions are valid for 6 months from date of issue except those for controlled drugs, which are valid for 13 weeks. An estimated 14.5% of prescriptions are not cashed in at all. Advise patients to destroy any unused prescriptions.

Reducing prescription fraud

Prescription theft and fraud is estimated to cost the NHS £15 million per year in England and Wales alone, so be vigilant to help reduce this (*Box 8.4*). All FP10 forms are numbered so you may have to sign out and account for all prescriptions you use.

Box 8.4 Reducing prescription fraud, tampering and theft

- Circle the quantity issued, or duration of course
- Rule a diagonal line though any blank space (computer will do so automatically)
- Countersign/initial any alterations
- Keep prescriptions out of sight (in consulting room, car, at reception)
- Do not leave patients unattended in your room where they have access to prescriptions
- Keep prescriptions in a locked drawer
- Take few prescriptions on visits

OPTIMISING PATIENT CONCORDANCE (COMPLIANCE)

Counsel your patient fully, particularly when starting new drugs (*Box 8.5*). Many packaged medicines have clear patient information leaflets but patients can be put off by comprehensive lists of possible side effects. You may need to put this into perspective for them.

Ensure your patient knows when and how to get repeat prescriptions (see *Repeat prescribing*) and when to come for review. Try to synchronise the due dates for each drug for those on multiple medications.

Box 8.5 Prescribing: counselling the patient

- Make clear:
  - the **purpose** of any medicine prescribed: is it a cure, symptom relief or prevention?
  - intended **duration** of treatment
  - arrange **review**
  - specific drug **monitoring** if appropriate
- Warn about
  - common **side effects**
  - significant **interactions**
  - potential for **dependency and tolerance**
  - other specific instructions
- Give written instructions for complex or changing regimes, e.g. reducing steroids
- Explain the practice repeat prescribing system

GENERIC PRESCRIBING

Prescribing by drug name rather than proprietary (brand) name is cost-effective, encourages consistency and is used as a measure of good prescribing. When presented with a generic prescription, pharmacists are not obliged to dispense a particular brand. You should explain to the patient that, on occasion, they may get a different looking drug or even a different name on the package but this should not affect their treatment. There are a few exceptions where it is medically necessary to prescribe a particular brand (*Box 8.6*).

Box 8.6   Exceptions to generic prescribing

Drugs with a narrow therapeutic index
- Lithium
- Cyclosporin

Modified release preparations (where different formulations give different bioavailability)
- Theophylline/aminophylline
- Diltiazem/nifedipine
- Anticonvulsants

Others
- Some oral contraceptives
- Some HRT preparations
- Combination medications (though generally not recommended anyway)

LONG TERM MEDICATION

To ensure safe prescribing for the many patients on long-term treatments, systematic reviews of medication and a foolproof repeat prescribing system are essential.

The medication review

This is an opportunity for a systematic review (*Box 8.7*) of the continuing need and safety of a patient's medicine. Effective medication reviews reduce the likelihood of medicine-related problems. The review is usually undertaken by the GP who best knows the patient, but can also be done by pharmacists, practice nurses and nurse practitioners with special training. Document the reviews in the medical record.

Box 8.7 Systematic approach to medication review

- Is the patient taking the medications you think they are taking?
- Review the original and continuing requirement for each drug and dose
  - Is it still appropriate?
  - Is it effective?
  - Is it the most cost-effective?
  - Is it being taken properly and are directions clear?
- Do they understand the purpose of the drugs?
- Are they happy to continue taking them?
- Ask specifically about:
  - Side effects (consider dose or drug changes if significant)
  - Alcohol intake
  - Other non-prescribed medications also taken (OTC, herbal and homeopathic treatments) and check interactions with these where known
- Institute relevant monitoring tests (including blood tests/BP)
  - ensure the patient understands the need for and frequency of these
  - chase up results and notify the patient of any necessary drug changes
- Clarify with the patient, with written instructions if necessary, and *document*
  - current regime, including new drugs and whether they are additions or substitutes
  - changes made at review
  - tests initiated with results
  - arrangement for next review

The nGMS contract* includes several quality markers dependent on medication reviews under both medicines management and chronic disease management (*Box 8.8*).

*See *Chapter 1: Working in general practice.*

Box 8.8 Examples of quality indicators dependent on the medication review

Medicines management 1 (2 points)
Details of prescribed medicines are available to the prescriber at each surgery consultation

Medicines management 5 (7 points)
A medication review is recorded in the notes in the preceding 15 months for all patients being prescribed repeat medications

Epilepsy (4 points)
The percentage of patients age 16 and over on drug treatment for epilepsy who have had a record of medication review in the previous 15 months

Patients under shared hospital and GP care

Department of Health guidelines stipulate that where care is shared between hospital and GPs the legal responsibility for prescribing lies with the doctor who signs the prescription

GPs often have to issue repeat prescriptions between hospital reviews so must ensure that there is written documentation and test results available from the hospital visits in the medical record before prescribing. Chasing up such information can be time-consuming, but is essential for patient safety and can be delegated to a member of staff. This is particularly important for drugs such as methotrexate and cyclosporin. Your PCO and hospital trust may have a 'shared care agreement' which sets out clear guidance for patients under shared care.

Essentially the prescriber is responsible for reviewing the treatment.

Medication changes should be recorded in the prescribing and medical record, and review dates amended when hospital letters are dealt with*. Enter the results of any drug monitoring tests to prevent duplication of these.

See Chapter 12: Paperwork, certificates and benefits.

Repeat prescribing

> *Repeat prescribing lends itself to mistakes, complaints and litigation so take rigorous clinical care when signing each prescription*

For patients on long-term medication the practice repeat prescribing system allows for the ordering of a script without the need for a face-to-face consultation each time. This has been revolutionised by computerisation: the computer also generates a list of repeat medication, which can be used for future requests and to remind patients of review dates.

Practice repeat prescribing policy

Repeat prescribing enables patients to obtain further supplies of an ongoing medicine without having to see the doctor. It accounts for 65–70% of GP prescriptions and 80% of GP prescribing costs.

All practices should have a written policy that is reviewed at least annually (*Box 8.9*). Familiarise yourself with the system so you can educate your patients accordingly. As the new person in the practice you're in a good position to identify and improve on any flaws in the current system.

Box 8.9   Key areas of the repeat prescribing protocol

Production – involves receiving requests and producing a prescription. Usually delegated to a practice receptionist

Management control – usually delegated to a trained staff member, comprising four elements:
1. Authorisation check
2. Compliance check
3. Review date – ensuring that every patient has a clear indicator of when therapy should be removed
4. Flagging – ensuring that each patient due for review is brought to the prescriber's attention

Clinical control – this is the doctor's, or other qualified prescriber's responsibility, and involves two tasks:
1. Authorisation – the decision that a repeat prescription is appropriate, the prescriber being satisfied that the drug is effective, well tolerated and still needed
2. Periodic review – a review of the patient and the medication to ensure that treatment is still effective, appropriate and well tolerated. The prescriber makes an informed decision as to whether to continue, change or stop medication

Adapted from Zermansky (1996)

Dealing with repeat prescription requests

Repeat prescriptions may be generated by a trained staff member but must be checked and signed by a doctor. As a new GP you should not be expected to sign the repeat prescriptions early on. You should be fully supervised when you first do this.

Check all the details on the prescription. If queries arise, access the medical record, discuss it with the partner who knows the patient well, or contact the patient in writing or by phone or ask them to make an appointment, in order to satisfy yourself that this prescription is appropriate. Don't sign if you are not sure.

If a review is due you may agree to prescribe a short supply but ensure the patient comes in for a review before the next prescription is issued.

Reception staff will be responsible for sending out prescriptions or leaving them for collection, usually in an indexed box.

You may be asked by reception staff to sign *ad hoc* repeat prescriptions for patients that 'can't wait', for example, going on holiday. Always adhere to good prescribing practice particularly when under pressure.

Repeat dispensing

This new initiative started development nationwide from 2004. It allows for patients with stable long-term conditions to be issued a single prescription that can be dispensed at intervals by a pharmacist of their choice. As the scheme develops it should include nurse and pharmacy prescribers. The system aims to reduce the need for GP practice generated 'repeats' and hopefully free up some GP time, as well as making use of pharmacists' skills and reducing waste.

Electronic transmission of prescriptions

Some practices are able to email prescriptions via protected pathways to designated pharmacies, reducing the need for patients to collect their scripts from the surgery.

PRESCRIBING IN SPECIFIC CASES

For the elderly

Take particular care with drug doses, reduce polypharmacy where possible and be alert to interactions. Try to avoid prescribing drugs with the potential for sedation and confusion. Prescribe very small quantities of drugs where you feel the drug is indicated but are concerned about possible adverse effects; review the patient and do not put the drug on 'repeat' e.g. for NSAIDs.

Use every opportunity to review medication, including on home visits. Encourage patients to return obsolete or date-expired medicines to their pharmacist. You may even remove them yourself but ensure you have the patient's permission.

Medication compliance aids, i.e. boxes divided into daily sections, can help to organise those on many medications, but access to the compartments may be difficult for patients with arthritis and drug or dose changes can be complicated to institute. The pharmacist or carer can fill the box on a regular basis but this in itself does not ensure compliance. The National Service Framework for Older People advises that patients on medication should have a medical review at least annually and 6-monthly if they are on more than four medications.

Written summary of changes and clear medication lists will improve patients' understanding of their medicines.

In pregnancy and breast feeding

Always check if a woman is, or might be, pregnant or breast feeding before prescribing and comply with advice in the *BNF* appendices. Manufacturers may advise against use in pregnancy and breast feeding because of lack of evidence on safe usage.

Anxiety often arises in women who may have taken drugs before realising they are pregnant. In such cases you may need to liaise with your hospital drug information service, the Regional and District Drug Information service (details in *BNF*) or even the manufacturers for advice.

For children

Prescribe according to any available paediatric formulary. You may need to use unlicensed medicines or licensed medicines for unlicensed purposes (see below) when prescribing in children. In such cases the parent/carer and child, where appropriate, should be fully informed and agreeable to the treatment.

Always check doses even for those drugs you think you know well. Most doses are given for age ranges or weight. In primary care you will rarely need to prescribe according to body surface area but there is a helpful conversion table at the back of the *BNF*. Get a colleague to double-check any dose calculations you make.

Advise parents of the indications for the medicine and of potential side effects, and remind them of safe storage of all medicines. Check for family history of severe penicillin allergy before prescribing for the first time.

Prescribe sugar-free formulations where available and avoid tablets or i.m. injections. The standard 5 ml medicine spoon is supplied where the dose is a multiple of 5 ml, otherwise the pharmacist will supply a medicine syringe. Syringes are particularly useful; advise parents to place the syringe between the cheek and gum margin, not directly on the tongue, with the child held at 45 degrees. Drugs shouldn't be added to bottles or feeds.

All prescriptions for children under 16 years, or under 18 years in full time education, are exempt from charges.

Antibiotics

> **Before prescribing antibiotics check for history of:**
> - allergy
> - pregnancy
> - breast feeding
> - interaction with current medication, e.g. warfarin and oral contraceptive pill

Follow local guidelines and be aware of local resistance patterns, e.g. for UTIs.

Be consistent in your refusal of antibiotics for the treatment of simple upper respiratory infections. Explain why they are not appropriate and back it up with written advice and OTC recommendations. This may take longer than issuing a prescription but it pays dividends in the long run. If necessary come to a compromise and issue a delayed prescription to be used should symptoms deteriorate within a specified time.

Prescribing over the phone

Prescriptions, with the exception of controlled drugs, can be telephoned through to a local pharmacist for collection by patients. This can be useful OOH or following a telephone consultation, but should only be undertaken if you are confident of your decision to initiate or continue treatment without the need for a face-to-face consultation. Send the written prescription to the pharmacist promptly. Be particularly diligent in documenting telephone directions for medication in the patient's notes.

Homeopathic and herbal medicines

Some of these treatments are available on FP10s. Unless you are specifically trained you may not be happy to prescribe so make this clear to the patient. Some herbal treatments have significant side effects and interactions, e.g. St. John's Wort and the combined oral contraceptive pill, so patients should not assume that natural treatments are harmless.

Controlled drugs

Marked CD in the *BNF*, controlled drugs include the familiar opiates and barbiturates. Controlled drug prescriptions must be written in full by hand in indelible ink. You must include:

- patient's name and address
- drug form

- dose, strength and the total quantity *in words and figures.*
- your address, signature and hand-written date

> **Computer-printed prescriptions for controlled drugs are not accepted unless prior arrangements have been made but you may write out the details on a blank FP10Comp. Prior arrangements are made for regular prescribers with approval from their PCO**

Pharmacists will telephone you if prescriptions are not completed accurately as they are not legally allowed to dispense unless the prescription is completed correctly. They often make allowances for mistakes on prescriptions for non-CD drugs, dispense the medication and then send back the prescription for correction.

The use of controlled drugs is governed by the Misuse of Drugs Act 1971 and the Misuse of Drugs Regulations amended 1985. Registered medical practitioners are allowed to 'possess and supply CDs when acting in a professional capacity' with the exception of schedule 1 drugs (*Box 8.10*). Doctors can be prosecuted for contravention of any of these regulations.

CDs must be kept in a locked compartment or receptacle and must be in a locked case if left in a locked car boot. The practice must keep a register to record supply and use of Schedule 2 CDs which the police or Home Office inspectors have a right to inspect every 2 years. If you keep Schedule 2 drugs in your bag you must have a separate register for this. Restocking your bag with a CD must be witnessed. Any destruction of a Schedule 2 CD must be witnessed by somebody authorised to do so, e.g. police officer, or PCO medical director.

Advise patients taking CDs and going abroad that they may require a specific licence from the Home Office, particularly if taking sizeable quantities of Schedule 2 and 3 drugs. Doctors carrying CDs abroad when accompanying patients may also need a licence.

Box 8.10   Controlled drug schedules (Misuse of Drug Regulations 1985)

Schedule 1   Cannabis/LSD – no therapeutic use (except research)
Schedule 2   Opiates and major stimulants
Schedule 3   Most barbiturates and some minor stimulants
Schedule 4   Benzodiazepines and anabolic steroids
Schedule 5   CDs combined with other drugs with minimal risk of abuse

Prescribing in the treatment of addiction

A special licence is required to prescribe heroin, cocaine or morphine in the treatment of addiction. For these, and methadone, the special blue prescription form FP10 MDA (GP10 in Scotland) should be used. Drug misusers no longer have to be registered with the Home Office but doctors should report cases to the local Drug Misuse Database (details in the *BNF*). Many practices will register drug-dependent patients for primary health care services, but may leave CD prescribing to the local Drug Dependency Unit.

*See *Chapter 1: Working in general practice.*

Prescribing for the treatment of addiction may be an enhanced service in the nGMS contract in your area*. Find out about local services. A session at the VTS may count towards your training to provide this service.

†See *Chapter 7: The consultation: survival tips for new GPs –* Manipulative patients.

Requests for drugs which you suspect are being used as alternatives to street drugs, typically benzodiazepines and opiates, can be difficult to manage†. Be guided by practice policy and ask for advice from your GP colleagues. Limit supplies to a few days only if you do agree to prescribe.

PAYING FOR MEDICINES

The patient

Prescriptions charges and exemptions

NHS prescriptions charges are set by government and increase most years. In 2003, 86% of all prescriptions issued were exempt from charges for medical, maternity and social reasons or on the grounds of age (*Box 8.11*). Pharmacists are increasingly vigilant in checking for evidence of eligibility for exemption from charges. All contraception is available free in the UK.

Medical and maternity exemption certificates are issued by the health authority following submission of form FP92A for medical conditions (*Box 8.12*) or FW8 for maternity exemption. These forms should be available in the surgery, completed by the patient, countersigned by the GP to confirm the condition, then forwarded to the health authority which issues the certificate.

Holders of medical exemption certificates are entitled to free medicines for all conditions not only the qualifying one. People who pay for more than five prescriptions every four months could save money by buying a pre-payment certificates (PPC); in 2004 a single prescription item cost £6.40 and a PPC for four months £33.40 and 12 months £91.80.

Over the counter medicines

Medicines are classified according to their availability to the public, generally on grounds of safety and tolerability (*Box 8.13*).

A large number of medicines are available OTC without prescription and it is always worth checking in the *BNF* when you prescribe. The Proprietary Association of Great Britain publishes an annual directory of such medicines.

Box 8.11 Prescription charge exemptions (see reverse of FP10 and form FP92A)

- Aged under 16 years
- Aged 16,17,18 years and in full time education
- Aged 60 years or over
- Holder of maternity exemption certificate
- Holder of medical exemption certificate (see below)
- Holder of prepayment certificate
- Holder of War Pension Exemption certificate
- Named on HC2 Charges certificate (entitled to help with health costs)
- Receiving:
  - Income Support
  - Income-based job seekers allowance
  - Full working families tax credit
  - Disabled person's tax credit
- Prescribed contraception

Box 8.12 Medical exemptions to prescription charges (FP92A form)

- Permanent fistula requiring continuous surgical drainage or appliance
- Epilepsy requiring continuous anti-convulsant therapy
- Diabetes mellitus (except diet-only controlled)
- Hypothyroidism
- Hypoparathyroidism
- Diabetes insipidus and other hypopituitarism
- Hypoadrenalism (including Addison's Disease) requiring substitution therapy
- Myasthenia gravis
- Continuing physical disability requiring help of another in order to go out

Box 8.13 Classification of medicines

PoM Prescription-only medication
P Pharmacy medicine – can be sold from pharmacists
GSL General Sales List – can be sold from shops and supermarkets

The pharmacist's role as health advisor continues to expand along with the list of P and OTC medicines, with the intention of encouraging self-care and reducing GP contacts. Patients exempt from charges or requiring a large quantity of non-prescription medicines may still request prescriptions.

Private prescriptions

Private prescriptions can only be issued to NHS patients for medication that cannot be prescribed on an FP10. Although some drugs available on FP10 may be cheaper on private prescription, GPs are not actually allowed to offer a private prescription alternative to their patients.

There are some prescription-only medicines in occasional use marked NHS in the *BNF* that cannot be prescribed on an NHS prescription. Where patients insist on such items and you feel the request is justified you can issue a private prescription either by computer or by hand on headed notepaper. Warn the patient that they will have to meet the full cost of the drug together with a pharmacist's dispensing fee so do not quote them the *BNF* price which is discounted for NHS use. Such drugs include:

- sildenafil (Viagra) for certain patient groups
- mefloquine (Lariam) for malarial prophylaxis (but not treatment of established cases)
- 'blacklisted' benzodiazepines

The NHS does not support the prescription of 'just in case drugs' such as antibiotics for foreign travel so you will need to prescribe privately if you agree to such requests. Patients who have been seen in the private sector and issued with a private prescription often ask for these to be converted to NHS prescriptions because their insurance does not cover drug costs. Discuss these occasional cases with one of the partners or other GPs before you prescribe.

Private prescriptions must include your professional address and GMC number. They can be used for initial stock drugs for your doctor's bag.

The Health Service

PACT — Prescribing Analysis and Cost data

Also known as SPA: Scottish Prescribing Analysis, or NIPPI: Northern Ireland Prescribing Prices Information.

PACT data are issued every 3 months to all GP principals by the Prescription Pricing Authority (PPA), which processes all dispensed NHS prescriptions. It provides summaries of GPs' individual and practice prescribing with information on the number of individual items and costs of the prescriptions dispensed (not issued). Local and national comparisons are provided together with data for the previous year.

Drugs are divided into the main six *BNF* therapeutic groups and the 20 leading prescriptions in the practice are identified. Practices can use this information to audit their prescribing.

Registrars should look through their trainer's PACT report in a tutorial. It will focus you on just how expensive drugs are and could be the basis of an MRCGP question.

Prescribing incentive schemes and prescribing indicators

Such schemes, run by some health authorities or PCOs, offer financial rewards to practices that fulfil certain 'good practice' prescribing criteria. With the introduction of nGMS and its quality indicators for prescribing some PCOs are no longer running these schemes. However, central prescribing indicators from bodies such as the Healthcare Commission may contribute to the star rating of the PCO areas on, e.g. prescribing patterns for benzodiazepines in their area.

Criteria for incentive schemes vary from region to region and from year to year but may include:

- high percentage of generic prescriptions
- low percentage of drugs known to be of limited therapeutic value
- ratio of bronchodilator : steroid inhalers prescribed
- NSAIDs prescribed from a locally approved list
- specified drug audits

Find out how your practice is involved so you can help and prescribe in line with local policy.

Some practices may hold an indicative budget for prescribing.

High cost medication

Some expensive specialist drugs are initiated in secondary care and GPs are then requested to continue prescribing them. GPs are not obliged to prescribe if they feel insufficiently experienced or are not willing to accept the clinical responsibility involved. This is particularly relevant for new specialist treatments.

Such treatments, which include fertility drugs, erythropoetin injections and enteral nutritional supplements, may cost thousands of pounds per patient per year. Your practice should have a policy on such prescribing based on locally approved shared care guidelines.

As a new GP it should not be up to you to decide whether or not to prescribe such drugs for patients. GPs asked to prescribe high cost medicines may need to seek advice from the prescribing advisor for their PCO as sometimes these items can be accounted for in the annual practice drug costs.

DRUG SAFETY ISSUES

Reporting adverse drug reactions

Remember to report adverse drug reactions (ADRs) to the Committee on Safety of Medicines using the Yellow Card system, at the back of the *BNF**.

*See Chapter 3: Working in the wider health service.

You should report on any therapeutic agent, including self-medication and herbal products:

- any reaction from new drugs (marked ▼ in the *BNF*)
- severe reactions from established drugs even if a well recognised reaction

Drug and product liability

Drug manufacturers are liable for their products under the Consumer Protection Act 1987 and patients can claim compensation from them should they suffer injury as a result of specific drug use. To avoid this liability falling to you as the GP, you must ensure the patient is fully informed about the appropriate use of the drug and keep adequate records documenting:

- date of prescription
- nature of illness
- tests to establish diagnosis
- quantity prescribed
- warnings of side effects
- problems experienced by the patient whilst taking the drug

You must document clearly the dose, batch number and expiry date of any drugs or injections you administer.

Prescribing unlicensed drugs

See Chapter 3: Working in the wider health service.

Drugs sold in the UK must have a Product Licence (marketing authorisation) granted by the Medicines and Healthcare Products Regulatory Agency*, which effectively confirms its effectiveness and safety and that it gives overall benefit.

There may be occasions when unlicensed drugs can be prescribed, or licensed drugs prescribed for indications outside their licence, e.g. for use in children. In such cases the patient must be fully informed that the drug is unlicensed and that all actions and side effects may not be known; document this in their notes. The drug may be available direct from the manufacturer on a 'named patient' only basis. This is not that common in general practice, and so you may need to seek advice from your colleagues and PCO pharmacy advisor.

DRUG INFORMATION SOURCES

WRITTEN MATERIAL	
The *BNF*	• Always use the current version: issued March and September • Read essential information in the front and appendices • Useful phone numbers inside front cover • Directory of drug manufacturers at the back • Electronic version available (eBNF)
Over the Counter Directory (Proprietary Association of Great Britain)	• Useful guide to save you from issuing prescriptions and to save money for your patients
Practice or PCO prescribing protocol or formulary	• Usually based on local prescribing guidance • Some exceptions are likely in practice
Drug and Therapeutics Bulletin	• Excellent and sensible evidence-based assessment of common therapeutic issues • Essential for day to day practice and MRCGP exam
MeReC bulletin	• Regular bulletin providing clear, concise evaluated information on medicines and prescribing-related issues • Published by National Prescribing Centre and funded by NICE • Available online at <u>www.npc.co.uk</u>
Drug Tariff	• NHS publication supplied to practices and pharmacists outlining all brands, clinical supplies and equipment available on the NHS • Useful for troublesome prescriptions for stoma bags, dressings, catheters, etc.
Paediatric reference – *Medicines for Children*	• Produced by RCPCH and Neonatal and Paediatric Pharmacists group and available online at <u>www.rcpch.ac.uk</u>

SERVICES AND ORGANISATIONS

Local pharmacists	• Usually happy to offer advice so keep telephone number handy
Hospital pharmacists and drug information service	• Helpful for queries particularly new drugs and interactions
PCO prescribing advisor	• Pharmacists employed by PCO to advise on local prescribing initiatives and difficulties • May offer support with practice audits
Regional and district drug information services	• Telephone numbers inside front cover of the *BNF* • Provide information on any aspect of drug use
Poisons Information Services	• Telephone number inside front cover of the *BNF* • First contact for acute overdose/poisoning incidents
Pharmacy at the Royal London Homeopathic Hospital	• Provide advice on homeopathic treatment including interactions with orthodox medicines
Drug companies	• Index of all manufacturers at back of *BNF* • Contact drug information departments for information on their individual products
National Prescribing Centre (NPC)	• NHS organisation promoting high quality cost-effective prescribing
Prescription Pricing Authority (PPA)	• NHS 'special health authority' • Provides feedback to prescribers, via PACT, and to Department of Health • Sets pricing arrangements for paying pharmacists and prescribing practices

SOURCES AND FURTHER READING

1. *British National Formulary,* www.bnf.org
2. Medicines and Healthcare Products Regulatory Agency, www.mhra.gov.uk
3. National Prescribing Centre, www.npc.co.uk
4. Prescription Pricing Authority, www.ppa.org.uk
5. National Electronic Library for Health, www.nelh.nhs.uk
6. Department of Health. *Health Information for Overseas Travellers.* HMSO, 2001 (The Yellow Book).
7. Department of Health. *Immunisation Against Infectious Disease.* HMSO, 1996 (The Green Book).
8. Royal College of Paediatrics and Child Health. *The use of unlicensed medicines or licensed medicines for unlicensed application in paediatric practice.* Policy statement from RCPCH and Neonatal and Paediatric Pharmacists Group Feb 2000, www.rcpch.ac.uk
9. National Prescribing Centre. *Saving time, helping patients – a good practice guide to quality repeat prescribing.* January 2004.
10. National Prescribing Centre. *A guide to good practice in the management of controlled drugs in primary care* (England). June 2004.
11. Zermansky A.G. Who controls repeats? *British Journal of General Practice* 1996; **46**: 643–7.

Chapter 9
Medical records and computers

INTRODUCTION

The medical record and computer are now integrally linked and GP packages are easy to learn and work with. General practice uses the computer for appointments, consultations, accessing information, coding of illness, and audit. A computer is indispensable for practices to ensure quality targets are hit and payments received under nGMS*. Most new GPs find the use of the computer in the consultation overwhelming initially, but become quite expert within a few weeks.

*See *Chapter 1: Working in general practice.*

The NHS Plan in 2000 made information technology a priority. The National Programme for Information Technology aims to set up a computer network which will allow health professionals including GPs, hospitals and pharmacists to share patient information. Ultimately patients should be able to access their own records from home. Other aims of the programme are to improve access to hospital outpatients[†] and a system to send electronic prescriptions to chemists.

†See *Chapter 10: Referrals – Choose and book.*

MEDICAL RECORDS

Whether in paper or electronic format, medical records are essential for continuity of patient care and medico-legal protection. Lost notes and crashed computers can slow up your surgery and impair good medical practice. NHS medical records belong to the health authority and not the GP or the patient. A doctor only has the legal right to use the notes to provide ongoing clinical care.

Documenting the consultation

> **Always write full and clear notes, particularly following a difficult consultation and ensure the date and time are documented**

GPs vary in the extent to which they record information and whether they complete records during or after the consultation. The test of an adequate medical record is that it enables you to reconstruct the consultation without reference to memory. Try to reduce the risk of forgetting important details by writing the notes as you see each patient and not to leave this until the end of the surgery, even if you are running late.

The acronym 'SOAP' can be used to structure the consultation findings in the notes (*Box 9.1*).

Documenting the consultation can take several minutes, but your note taking will become slicker with experience and time pressure, but should always include a sensible minimum of information.

Box 9.1   Documenting consultations: S.O.A.P.

S	Subjective	What the patient tells you / history
O	Objective	Your examination findings
A	Assessment	Your working diagnosis / problem title
P	Plan	Your management: investigations, referrals, treatment and follow up

You should:

- document relevant negative findings to show you actively considered them
- avoid the excessive use of abbreviations
- record any health promotion advice you give – this is essential for audit and nGMS*
- document all consultations including phone consultations, discussions with hospital specialists about patients, and opinions you give to health professional colleagues
- never write derogatory comments about the patient, their relatives or colleagues

*See *Chapter 1: Working in general practice.*

Taking care of medical records

Respect patients' medical records! Don't leave letters or paper notes lying around where other patients could read them or leave your computer screen showing details of your previous patient.

Reception staff should all receive training in the importance of confidentiality, accurate filing and the use of a reliable tracer system.

Disclosure of medical information from the records to a third party is covered in detail in *Chapter 21: Guidance for good professional practice – Disclosing medical information.*

Amending medical records

Records should only be amended if the information is inaccurate, misleading or incomplete. If you need to make changes then make it clear you are doing so by adding a note which you should date and initial with a reason for the change or late entry. Don't make any changes that could later be interpreted as an intention to mislead. Should a patient disagree with an entry then it can be amended (not removed) with a dated statement from the patient to that effect. Computer programmes are able to trace changes and deletions made to patients' notes so ensure you always log on correctly and don't allow others to use your terminal without changing to their username and password first. Lock your computer screen if you leave the room.

Patients cannot dictate what information goes into their notes; it is up to the doctor to decide what is relevant for the clinical care of the patient. You may need to explain this to patients who ask you to omit certain information from their notes. If you do enter the information and are subsequently challenged by the patient then be prepared to justify your decision.

Future disclosure of clinical information to a third party, particularly insurers, can have adverse implications for the patient.

Patient access to medical records

Under the Data Protection Act (1998) patients are allowed access to their entire medical record, unless:

- the doctor feels disclosure of information would cause *serious* harm to their mental or physical health, or
- information about a third party would be revealed without their consent

If a patient asks to see their records there and then and you have concerns about this, discuss this with one of your colleagues or the practice manager. Although the Act does not give patients the right to inspect their records straight away, if both the note-holder and patient agree, and the above exemptions don't apply, then you may let them have immediate access.

Bear in mind the following points that should be explained to patients wishing to see their records:

- requests should be made in writing to the practice
- no reason is needed
- the practice must supply the patient, or someone authorised on their behalf, with copies of the relevant notes within 40 days of the request unless there are good reasons to deny access (see above)
- explanations must be given if information isn't easy to understand, e.g. medical abbreviations, either by appointment or in writing
- all written requests for access to notes should be date-stamped and kept with copies of the information disclosed, separate from the notes

The Data Protection Act also covers issues on protecting patient information.

COMPUTERS

GP practices are all computerised to a greater or lesser extent. Many practices are now paperless or more accurately paper-light. The computer is used for medical records, appointments, patient information services, referrals, audit, practice book-keeping and accounts and is vital in a modern primary care service (*Box 9.2*).

Box 9.2 Potential uses of the computer in general practice

Look at the main menu on your computer package

Patient management
- Medical records
- Past history
- Medical summary including new patient registration check
- Consultation entries
- Results
- Chronic disease management templates
- Diary due dates
- Prescribing
- Word processing
- Referral letters
- Scanned documents, e.g. letters from the hospital
- Clinical protocols and guidelines

Practice management
- Appointments system
- Practice profile/demographics
- Practice accounts

Databases
- Practice phone directory
- *eBNF*
- Patient information leaflets
- Medical decision support software, e.g. Mentor, Prodigy

Communications
- Internal and external e-mail
- 'Links' to hospital pathology lab./radiology
- Links to health authority for claims
- NHSnet
- Internet
- Intranet

Research and education
- Patient searches
- Audit
- Statistical analysis
- Medline/other search
- Online journals/circulars

GP software packages are available with training, upgrades and help-lines. These allow you to enter data as free text and also in response to fixed prompts, which are coded and so can be easily traced for audit and research purposes.

Training

As entering information on the computer during surgeries will really slow you down to start with, make sure you have some IT training in your induction period. Most GP packages have a 'play' mode to practice on.

Find out who are the IT leads in the practice as they will be the ones to turn to when the system crashes, the printers don't work or you've pressed the wrong button.

Establish the minimum computer-use expected of you. This will expand with experience and after a few months you should be familiar with day to day use, searches, prescribing and audit.

The computer in the consultation

Make sure you exit your last patient's notes before calling in your next patient. Don't let the consultation be dominated by your computer.

Positioning your computer

Ideally your screen should be directly ahead of you. If this is not possible then the right-handed should have the computer on the right hand-side of the desk and the patient to the left, *vice versa* for the left handed. Don't let the computer sit as a barrier between you and the patient. Your forearms should be horizontal and your eyes the same height as the top of the screen. Wrists should be kept straight. Neither you nor the screen should face windows or bright lights.

Data entry

Try to enter numbers as you take them, e.g. weight, BMI and peak flow, even if you do most of your typing when the patient has left. With experience you'll be able check medication, due-dates for smears and vaccinations, and past history as you go. You should develop familiarity with frequently used codes (see below).

If your practice uses both hand-written and computer records ensure that some reference is made of the consultation in both.

Computer templates act as useful prompts, particularly for chronic diseases, health checks and contraception. Templates also make sure you enter information in codes (see below) consistent with other members of the practice, allowing for accurate audits.

Coding systems

Medical coding systems, e.g. 'Read codes' are in use throughout the NHS and allow clinical data to be entered according to a hierarchy system. As data are entered you are offered a choice of codes from fixed clinical labels. There may be more than one label for the same diagnosis so establish those most commonly used in your practice. Aim to use the 'highest' code. Accurate coding is essential for future searches and audit.

Prescribing on the computer

Always check you are in the correct patient's file before prescribing. Check all the information on the printed prescription before signing it

Computers are extremely useful in prescribing*:

*See *Chapter 8: Prescribing.*

- computer-generated scripts are legible and instantly recorded
- current and past medication are easily traced
- generic equivalents are easily found
- recorded allergies and significant interactions are flagged up.

You should be able to generate NHS or private prescriptions, prescribe for future issue and record anything issued by hand or a third party. A copy of the repeat medication list should be in the hand-held records. This right-hand section of the FP10Comp can also be used to let the patient know about medication review reminders, vaccination invitations and changes to practice details.

'Links'

Your practice may be electronically linked to:

- *The pathology/radiology/respiratory function services* which speeds up the return of results. Clarify the practice policy for acting on and filing both computer and paper results†.
- *Referral systems* which gives GP practices direct access to hospital outpatient and day-case surgery appointments. This is currently in various stages of development throughout the UK regions.

†See *Chapter 11: Investigations and results* – Linked results.

Databases

Systems usually have the scope for a practice telephone directory; use this to access, add and edit information on local NHS, private and voluntary sector services and contact numbers for staff.

Medical decision support packages such as Mentor and Prodigy should be available as well as regularly updated patient information leaflets. You can also direct patients to information websites such as www.patients.co.uk and www.besttreatments.co.uk.

Communications

You should be provided with an NHS email address to receive DOH, PCO, practice, and patient information. Email can turn into yet another in-tray demanding your attention. The scope for connecting to the outside world is huge. The National Electronic Library for Health (NELH) provides clinicians with updated information for use in clinical decision making. It provides access to other sites, e.g. *Drugs and Therapeutics Bulletin* and health databases. Registrars should consider arranging some VTS training in how to get the best out of the internet. Use our website address list as a starting point*.

See Appendix 1: Useful websites.

Protecting patient information

The Data Protection Act (1998) governs the processing of information held in health, education and social services records, both manual and computerised. Processing includes obtaining, storing and disclosing information (*Box 9.3*).

Practices must have a Data Protection Officer who is responsible for information handling and must register details and security measures with the Data Protection Commissioner. It is a criminal offence not to be registered under the Act.

Box 9.3   Data protection principles (Data Protection Act 1998)

1. Data must be:
   - relevant to the purpose for which they were obtained
   - accurate
   - kept up to date

2. Appropriate security measures to protect data must be in place

3. Guidance is given on:
   - sensitive information on race, ethnic origin, physical and mental health and sexual life
   - material used for research purposes

SOURCES AND FURTHER READING

1. National Programme for Information Technology in the NHS, www.npfit.nhs.uk
2. National Electronic Library for Health, www.nelh.nhs.uk
3. www.patient.co.uk
4. www.besttreatments.co.uk
5. Knight B. *Legal Aspects of Medical Practice*, Churchill Livingstone, 5th edition, 1992.
6. Panting G. *et al. Medical Records.* Medical Protection Society, 1999.
7. GMC. *Confidentiality: Protecting and providing information.* GMC, 2000.
8. DOH. *The Data Protection Act 1998 Protection and use of patient information.* DOH, 2003.
9. Health and Safety Executive. *Working with VDUs*, www.hse.gov.uk
10. RCGP information sheet. *General Practice Computerisation.* March 2003.

Chapter 10
Referrals

INTRODUCTION

GPs are obliged to arrange referrals for their patients to other services when this is clinically indicated. With waiting times for outpatients and operations continually in the public and political eye, we tread a fine line between serving our patients best without overloading secondary care. GPs should have access to information on local services on their desktop and can now book appointments online during the consultation.

Individual GP referral patterns vary due to both patient and doctor factors, such as difficulty tolerating uncertainty. Paradoxically, GPs with particular experience of a specialty are more, not less, likely to refer to it.

The introduction of indicative budgets for practices, or groups of practices, enhanced services, GPs with a special interest, and clinical assessment services, aim to reduce the number of patients referred from primary to secondary care.

You are responsible for the referrals you make and so must be confident of the qualifications of those you refer to. If you refer to a non-medical practitioner, e.g. an osteopath, then make sure they are members of a statutory regulatory body.

Don't be surprised if as a new GP you refer a lot initially. You are expected to practice only within the limits of your expertise, so seek help if you are out of your depth rather than opting for a best guess.

Registrars may find inviting consultants in the specialities in which they lack confidence to the VTS half-day release course, or you could arrange to sit in on their outpatient clinics*.

*See *Chapter 16: Educational aspects of the GP registrar year* – Specialist hospital outpatients.

WHERE TO REFER?

Seek advice or arrange a tutorial to find out how to refer patients to frequently used local services (*Box 10.1*). It will sometimes be unclear to which specialty you should refer.

Useful information sources:

- Trainer, GP colleagues, practice secretary
- Directory of secondary care services available locally (this will be available online)
- Local and national referral guidelines, e.g. NICE
- Local hospital circulars on waiting times

EMERGENCY REFERRALS

Arranging urgent hospital assessment for patients can be time-consuming and is particularly disruptive mid-surgery.

Box 10.1 Directing your referrals

Identify:

Services offered within the practice and alternatives outside the practice:
- IUDs
- joint injections
- minor surgery
- drug dependency services

Age cut-off for services for:
- paediatric
- adolescent
- adult
- care of the elderly services

Gestation cut-off for gynaecology versus obstetrics (usually 20 weeks)

Specialty accepting 'grey area' diagnoses such as:
- pyelonephritis
- back pain

Referral criteria for tertiary services:
- fertility
- plastic surgery

Sexual and reproductive medicine services:
- family planning
- termination
- early pregnancy unit
- genitourinary medicine services

One-stop diagnostic clinics:
- haematuria
- post-menopausal bleeding

Talking therapy services – NHS and other agencies:
- counselling
- cognitive behavioural therapy
- psycho-sexual
- psychotherapy

Allied health professionals – may have special forms
- physiotherapy
- OT
- foot health

Social services
- accept referrals from individuals, carers and health professionals

Other services
- palliative care
- drug and alcohol teams
- intermediate care

Getting your patient accepted

Some hospitals have a centralised system or a nursing manager accepting calls for emergency GP referrals. Alternatively speak to the on-call team.

If the problem isn't straightforward you are likely to have to 'sell' the case. Spend a few moments collecting your thoughts and clinical findings before you contact the hospital team; remember you may be more experienced than the doctor accepting the call. You only need to have done a clinical assessment sufficient to decide whether the patient requires referral. Avoid unpleasant examinations unless they alter your decision to refer, as they will inevitably be repeated by the admitting team.

If the on-call doctor refuses a referral without good reason or fails to offer an alternative management plan acceptable to you, let them know you will discuss the case with their consultant. This is rarely needed, but the consultant will invariably accept the patient on behalf of their team.

Sending the patient in

Send a hand-written or typed referral letter with the patient or fax a letter to A&E marked for the attention of the admitting team. Attach a computer-generated patient summary with personal details, past history and medication list and ensure a copy of any letter is kept in the patient's notes. Give the patient clear instructions as to where to go, which team is expecting them and whether they can expect to be admitted. Don't attempt a guess at how soon they will be seen. You may find patients reluctant to be referred for possible admission so you may have to be persuasive (see below).

Arranging an ambulance

If the patient is seriously ill or has no other safe way of travelling to hospital then arrange an ambulance (*Box 10.2*).

Keep a record of the GP priority ambulance line for whenever you are visiting or on call. If you delegate organising the ambulance to reception staff, give them full patient details for ambulance control. You will be given a reference number, which should be documented in the patient's medical record, together with the time of the request, so delays can be chased up.

In some conditions, e.g. a bad asthma attack, it may be safer for the patient to wait for an ambulance than to be taken in their own car and you should stay with the patient until the ambulance arrives.

If it's clear from a phone consultation that a 999 ambulance is needed, arrange this and try to get to the patient yourself if you can. If you can't make it before the ambulance still let A&E or the specialist team know that the patient is on their way.

Box 10.2 Arranging an ambulance

999
- For suspected MI, severe SOB, unconsciousness, potentially life threatening or other serious condition

Within the hour
- For moderate/severe pain

Within 2 hours
- Most other conditions

Details for ambulance control*
- Phone number you are calling from
- Your name and contact details
- Patient's contact phone number
- Latest time of arrival at hospital
- Address for pick up with nearest road junction or landmark
- Patient name, age, sex
- Diagnosis
- Any special instructions, e.g. oxygen
- Details of patient escort
- Destination

*Adapted from *Information for GPs and Clinicians*, London Ambulance Service, March 1998.

Patients refusing emergency referral

Some patients will refuse urgent referral when you consider it necessary. Explain why you advise referral for an assessment and that they can always refuse admission if it is offered.

Try to find out why they are refusing, e.g. hospital phobia, death of their spouse in hospital or fear of long A&E wait, and try to address their fears. You have a duty to explain why you feel it necessary to refer them and make clear the possible consequences of their refusal. Be honest about possible outcomes of their refusal but don't scaremonger. If they still refuse then respect their decision, document it fully in the notes and arrange the best alternative care (*Box 10.3*). If the patient is competent* you cannot insist they accept referral or admission.

If they are not competent, e.g. acute confusional state, you may act in their best interests and refer, but be prepared to justify this[†]. Restraint and tranquillising drugs may be used but only in exceptional circumstances.

If the patient is mentally ill and a danger to themselves or others a mental health section may be required[†].

*See *Chapter 21: Guidance for good professional practice –* Competence.

[†]See *Chapter 21: Guidance for good professional practice –* Treating incompetent adults.

[‡]See *Chapter 22: Clinical issues with legal stipulations –* The Mental Health Act and acutely mentally ill patient.

Private emergency admissions

Though some private hospitals do have a centralised admission system for urgent referrals you usually have to contact a willing private specialist, hospital and private ambulance service.

Encourage patients in emergency situations to use an NHS facility. Reassure them that the NHS handles emergencies quickly and that private hospitals may be less well equipped to deal with some emergencies. Patients can always negotiate a private transfer with their consultant once they are over the acute stage.

For less serious conditions that need admission and the patient is adamant they only want a private admission, write a referral letter and ask the patient to make their own admission arrangements by contacting a private hospital and specialist themselves.

NON-EMERGENCY REFERRALS

Referring to the Primary Health Care Team

Referrals to district nurses, health visitors, midwives or social services can be done in person, by letter or *pro-forma*, over the phone or via a referral book. These should always be afforded the same respect as other referrals. Make clear the reason for your referral and state exactly what you want from the service, e.g. continence assessment, ulcer dressing, or just 'assessment'. Document in the patient notes any verbal referral, copy or scan in any referral form completed with dates. You should receive feedback in practice meetings with members of the PHCT*.

*See *Chapter 2: Working in the team.*

Outpatient referrals

The majority of your referrals will be for secondary care outpatient appointments. These referrals can be made in writing or online depending on the services in your area. It's useful to discuss some cases with the relevant team, particularly for unclear problems. The online system should allow you to have an email conversation with consultants about patients and whether or not to refer and what the urgency is.

Chasing up lost referrals and appointments should be delegated to the patient or practice staff.

Make it clear to patients that they should come back to you should their symptoms deteriorate as you may be able to arrange an earlier appointment. Ask those whose conditions have improved to cancel their appointments.

Your practice may have guidelines for referrals to secondary care, especially if they hold an indicative budget for this.

'Choose and book'

From the end of 2005 all patients should be able to choose the place, time and date of their initial outpatient appointment. The 'Choose and book' system involves online referrals by GPs to a range of hospitals and services. Patients can decide in the GP consultation as to where and when they want to go and they can be given their appointment before leaving the surgery. Alternatively they can go away with a personal booking number and password and consider their choices. They can then make the appointment themselves online or via a telephone call to the local Booking Management Service (BMS). This was not in place when this book went to press, and implementation of 'Choose and book' may vary around the country.

Clinical assessment services

At the time of going to press PCOs are beginning to set up Clinical Assessment Services (CAS) to try and control demand on secondary care services. These vary from a clinician-led paper triage of referral letters, to clinical assessment of patients by a GP with a special interest (GPwSI) or an allied health professional. The health professional will manage and discharge some patients, and forward the rest on to secondary care services. These services are in their infancy, but may offer an opportunity for GPs to gain experience or training in a particular specialty.

Referrals to allied health professionals

Physiotherapy, occupational therapy, midwifery and talking therapies may be offered as hospital and community services. They often have forms and specific guidelines for referrals. These services may be one of the choices of the 'Choose and book' system for some conditions, e.g. joint pains.

Private referrals

Use recommendations from your GP colleagues, consultants you have worked with, and the local NHS hospital specialists who work privately. Find out who provides local private physiotherapy, osteopathy and radiology services.

Practices have different systems and may post the referral letter or leave it for the patient to collect. The patient then contacts the specialist's secretary to arrange their own appointment.

Those with private health insurance should contact their insurance company for prior agreement for the referral and a claim form.

Those who wish to pay their own way do not need your 'blessing'. Strictly speaking they do not need a referral letter either, although it is good practice to write one.

Practices may charge a fee for private referral letters and completing claim forms for private insurance.

Complementary therapy referrals

With the increasing popularity of complementary therapies, GPs are increasingly expected to advise and refer. There are very few NHS osteopathy and acupuncture services and so most patients will need to pay for these services. If you do not know what the therapy involves or doubt its effectiveness then say so. You may provide patients with contact details so they can do their own research but make it clear you are not formally recommending the treatment or referring them. Osteopaths and chiropracters have their own regulatory body, and it's reasonable to rely on membership of these as evidence of training.

GPRs may invite complementary practitioners to talk at VTS half-day release courses to inform you about their therapies.

REFERRAL LETTERS

Though many referrals are now done online, there is often still a need for the old-fashioned referral letter. Well-summarised medical records should speed up the referral letter process as personal details, past medical history, medication and allergies can be downloaded from the patient's computerised record. You may want to tidy or update the computer record before your referral letter is done*.

*See Chapter 9: Medical records and computers.

Find out how referrals are typed in your practice and ensure there is a clear system for all letters to be kept in the medical records.

> **Make clear to your secretary the priority of all your referrals:**
>
> * **emergency** = **now**
> * **urgent** = **within 24 hours**
> * **routine** = **anything longer**

> **Patients with a possible diagnosis of cancer should be referred the same day and see a specialist within 2 weeks**

Reduce your paperwork by identifying the services that allow self-referral, e.g. social services, drug dependency, podiatry for the elderly. Referral *pro formas* may be available on your practice computer system.

Aim to do all your letters after each surgery while the problem is fresh in your mind. Otherwise catch up at least weekly.

Dictation is usually quickest but takes practice so use our guide initially (*Boxes 10.4* and *10.5*) though some GPs will write by hand or even type themselves, especially for emergency referrals. Your practice should provide you with a dictaphone and you should keep a spare tape in your room.

Box 10.4   Referral letter: essential contents

- Be concise but complete
- **Ensure a copy is kept in the notes**
- Patient's problem as a title before the text e.g. *Asymptomatic inguinal hernia*
- Reason for the referral, e.g.
  - hospital involvement essential
  - second opinion (at yours or the patient's request)
  - exclusion of a serious diagnosis
  - diagnostic uncertainty
  - treatment failure
- Brief and relevant history
- Any treatment tried to date
- Results of relevant investigations
- What the patient has been told, especially in cases of contentious diagnoses, e.g. 'I have explained to the patient that MS is a possible diagnosis'
- Request for transport and translators if needed

Downloadable from patient record:
- Full patient details and current phone number – **confirm these with patient**
- NHS number and hospital number if known
- Relevant and significant past medical history
- Current regular medication
- Known allergies

Consultants prioritise outpatient appointments on the basis of your letter

Box 10.5 Dictation tips

- Start the tape with an introduction such as 'Dr X's letters on Tuesday 4th May'
- Dictate URGENT letters on a separate tape and clearly mark as such
- Speak clearly and slowly
- Spell difficult medical and other long words
- Give clear grammatical directions: 'Full stop. New paragraph'.
- Make the addressee clear: 'Dear Dr' or a specific consultant/hospital/speciality
- Stipulate:
  - NHS or private
  - Urgent or routine
  - For faxing, sending or collection by patient
  - Whether a fee has been/will be incurred
- Clear instructions on enclosures, i.e. copies of results/old letters/invoices
- Request that important words are highlighted or in bold (**'URGENT', '? Rectal carcinoma'**)
- Don't put too many letters on one tape

Correct typing errors and aim to sign all your own letters before they go out. Signing outgoing letters for absent partners can reveal different styles, problems and consultant preferences. Overall practice referral data should be available from the PCO. Registrars should spend a tutorial reviewing their own referrals for a week to reflect on their appropriateness and style.

Some practices have voice recognition packages for referral letters or may use distant typing services. Letters are dictated into a computer package, anonymised with an identifying code and emailed to a distant typist and emailed back when done.

SOURCES AND FURTHER READING

1. GMC. *Good Medical Practice* 3rd Edition. GMC, 2001.
2. GMC. *Seeking Patients' Consent: the Ethical Considerations*. GMC, 1998.
3. NICE. *Referral Advice. A Guide to Appropriate Referral from General to Specialist Services*, 2001. www.nice.org.uk
4. London Ambulance Service NHS Trust. *Information for GPs and Clinicians* London Ambulance Service, www.londonambulance.nhs.uk
5. www.chooseandbook.nhs.uk

Chapter 11
Investigations and results

INTRODUCTION

GPs spend a lot of time organizing, explaining and checking the results of investigations for patients. Try and develop a systematic approach so this does not become too burdensome for you.

Remember:

*See Chapter 21: Guidance for good professional practice – Understanding consent.

- You should always have a patient's informed consent before undertaking any investigation*.
- The practice should have a documented, fail-safe system for processing all results and you should understand this.
- Follow-up of all abnormal results is essential and the responsibility of the requesting doctor or doctor clearly delegated the task.

ORGANISING INVESTIGATIONS

Find out from your colleagues where most of the commonly requested GP investigations are carried out locally (see *Box 11.1*). There is currently a big push for more near-patient investigations so be aware of local service provisions and changes.

Take care when dealing with specimens, as lost or unlabelled specimens generate additional work for you and inconvenience for your patient (*Box 11.2*).

Box 11.1   Investigation services for GP patients

Find out what you are able to request and what can only be requested from secondary care

- Phlebotomy
- Paediatric
  - phlebotomy
  - bag urine collection
- Simple radiology/ultrasound
- Specialist radiology, e.g. CT, MRI
- ECG
- Echocardiography
- Exercise and ambulatory ECG
- Endoscopy
- *H. pylori* breath testing
- Bone density scanning
- Glucose tolerance tests
- Retinal screening
- Semen analysis

GPs usually delegate taking blood except when with an acutely ill patient or on a home visit.

Ideally practices should keep a record of all specimens sent from the practice to check that all results are received. Keep a record of particularly important tests you request. Document clearly if you have advised patients to come back for results or will let them know if there are any problems with the results. Make sure you stick to what you said.

Urgent requests

Pathology

Urgent requests should be phoned ahead to the laboratory or bleep the duty technician. Ask for the results to be phoned or faxed back the same day. Mark the request form 'urgent' and ensure practice contact details are clear. You may need to organize special transport for the specimen. Make arrangements with another doctor to chase up results later if you are not going to be around.

Radiology/ultrasonography

Telephone the department directly for urgent radiology. Same-day gynaecology ultrasound scans to exclude ectopic pregnancy may be arranged in specialized early pregnancy units. Other imaging may require specific discussion with the on-call radiologist. You may need to fax the request form.

Housebound patients

On home visits take any necessary bloods yourself, otherwise ask the practice or district nurse to do this. If an elderly patient needs several investigations as well, such as an ECG and CXR, then consider referring them to a day hospital or out-patient service for a full work-up, for which transport can be arranged.

Uncommon tests

Check with the pathology laboratory the bottle or container required for unusual or unfamiliar tests you request. Make this clear on the request form if you are not taking the sample yourself.

Some tests may only be undertaken with appointments, e.g. semen analysis, or by specialist centres, e.g. genetic screening, so find out from colleagues or the relevant laboratory. You will occasionally be asked to take bloods for a patient as part of a research project or for a private medical. A kit will usually be supplied and sent back in the post. Check if there is a fee payable.

Patients may request tests that are unusual in daily general practice, e.g. selenium levels or 'allergy tests', or have been recommended by a complementary practitioner. Try to discover any underlying worries which may reveal the patient's fears but do not agree to investigations if you will not be able to interpret the results or there is no evidence base or clinical indication.

Beware the patient who seems to want 'testing for everything'. There is usually an underlying agenda, which you will need to unravel.

Patients refusing investigations

Patients sometimes opt out of investigations, preferring to wait and see, or decide not to have them done simply because they get better.

Difficulties arise when patients actively refuse investigations which you consider clinically important. Approach these situations as you would patients refusing referral*. Ask them why they are declining. Dislike of needles can be overcome using local anaesthetic, cream or psychotherapy. Explain fully your reasons for requesting the investigation and the consequences of not having it.

*See Chapter 10: Referrals – Patients refusing emergency referral.

If you feel they are competent to refuse[†] then respect their wishes, document your explanation and their refusal in the medical record and arrange alternative management.

†See Chapter 21: Guidance for good professional practice – Refusal of consent.

Difficult situations include the elderly confused patient who may have a treatable cause for their mental state and those with severe learning disabilities whom you suspect have a physical problem yet are unable to co-operate. You may need to act in their 'best interests'[‡]. Seek advice from your GP colleagues.

‡ See Chapter 21: Guidance for good professional practice.

Private tests

There may be a local private pathology and radiology service for patients who do not want to use the NHS service.

WHICH INVESTIGATIONS

GP investigations will be for diagnostic, screening or monitoring purposes though they can also be used, with discretion, to buy time and exclude serious pathology when you are unsure how to manage an unclear presentation*.

Be wary of over-investigating as this is costly and can encourage increased patient expectations. Limit your investigations to those which will help your management. Nursing staff may generate investigations and you may need to act upon these results too.

*See *Chapter 7: The consultation: survival tips for the new GP.*

Monitoring chronic conditions and drug treatment

There is little consensus on the exact frequency of investigations and review for long-term diseases or drug monitoring. Be guided by evidence-based guidelines, the *BNF*, your colleagues and hospital specialists. Computer prompts and diary due dates can help ensure patients are followed up.

Check opportunistically in consultations if repeat investigations are required, or leave messages and pathology request forms for patients when collecting their repeat prescriptions.

Before signing a script for a drug that needs monitoring, clarify and document clearly who is responsible for monitoring tests for those patients under shared specialist and GP care[†]. Update the medical record with relevant test results from hospital letters[‡].

†See *Chapter 8: Prescribing – Patients under shared GP and hospital care.*

‡See *Chapter 12: Paperwork, certificates and benefits.*

Screening tests

Screening is an important part of general practice, and a big topic for the MRCGP.

Given the uncertainties involved in some screening tests and the potentially serious consequences of a positive test, you must be sufficiently informed to counsel patients adequately (see *Box 11.3*). This is a useful topic for a clinical meeting or VTS teaching afternoon.

Box 11.3   Counselling patients for screening investigations

Explain:

- the purpose of the screening
- the likelihood of false positive and negatives
- any uncertainties and risks involved in the process
- significant medical, social or financial implications of the screening
- follow up plans

You should inform patients of how and when they should receive the results of any screening test. Your practice should have a fail-safe system for processing cervical smear results so find out how this works. Breast screening is usually organized by the health authority or PCO.

Antenatal screening tests

Screening in pregnancy can generate enormous anxiety and raises many difficult questions. Clarify:

- what is offered to women at your local antenatal service
- who is responsible for chasing up the basic antenatal screening tests (GP or midwives)
- how the woman can access her results

There are many different antenatal screening tests, e.g. nuchal fold, quadruple test. Find out exactly what is offered locally and ensure your knowledge is sufficiently up to date to counsel women effectively on the pros and cons of each test. Use written information on the statistics of risk and of procedures such as amniocentesis. Give the woman and her partner an opportunity to ask questions.

DEALING WITH RESULTS

It is your responsibility to ensure that you have seen and acted on results of all the tests you request

Your practice will have a system for processing all incoming results, both paper and electronic versions and for patients to access their results.

Paper results should be date-stamped and directed to the requesting doctor. They may also be stamped with a variety of options for your action (*Box 11.4*).

Box 11.4 Practice results stamp instructions

- Seen by Dr ......
- Tell patient normal
- File
- Pull notes for Dr ......
- Ask patient to phone Dr ......
- Ask patient to make appointment
- Needs repeat, form left for collection
- Ask patient to collect prescription
- Other

Sign or initial all your results. If you are away then make sure that someone sees your results in your absence.

Results taken over the phone should be documented in the medical record and marked as such in case errors occurred in transcribing. Make sure you also see the paper or electronic version.

Include relevant test results in your outpatient referral letters.

Linked results

If your practice is electronically linked to the local laboratory results will be sent to the practice on secure IT links and once approved filed directly in the patient's computer medical record.

Abnormal results

Straightforward

Simple abnormal results such as confirmed UTI or positive throat swab should be easy to deal with:

- check current treatment in the medical record
- if treatment is needed contact the patient by telephone or letter depending on urgency.
- arrange management such as prescriptions, or further investigations and leave forms at reception
- document your actions in the medical record

Patients should be invited in for an appointment for abnormal screening tests that may have significant implications such as haemoglobinopathies or markedly elevated cholesterol levels.

The laboratory may add a helpful interpretation or suggest an action such as 'Notify'* or suggest rubella vaccination.

*See *Chapter 22: Clinical issues with legal stipulations –* Notifiable diseases.

Seriously abnormal results

Dangerously abnormal results, such high INR or elevated potassium and less acute, but serious abnormalities such as possible lung cancer, will usually be phoned through to you. Consider your management options before contacting the patient[†].

†See *Chapter 7: The consultation: survival tips for the new GP –* Breaking bad news.

Mildly abnormal or 'unclear' results

These can present problems, particularly if you are dealing with the results for a patient you do not know well. Review the medical records and arrange a repeat test if necessary to see the trend of the abnormality and ask for advice from your GP or specialist colleagues.

SOURCES AND FURTHER READING

1. GMC. *Seeking Patients' Consent: the Ethical Considerations,* GMC, 1998.
2. UK National Screening Committee, www.nsc.nhs.uk

Chapter 12
Paperwork, certificates and benefits

INTRODUCTION

The volume of GP paperwork has increased dramatically over the last decade due in part to increased NHS bureaucracy and patient and third party demands, some of which can seem ridiculous.

As a new GP you will be unlikely to have the volume of a partner's paperwork but good habits for dealing with paperwork early on will stand you in good stead for the future. Dealing with the post of an absent partner for a week or two can be a good eye-opener as to what they have to contend with on a daily basis (*Box 12.1*).

Box 12.1   Making sense of incoming mail

Patient-related
- Pathology and radiology results
- Letters from secondary care and allied health professionals
- Communications from patients including prescriptions and referral requests
- Statutory and private forms for completion
- Requests for letters, e.g. 'fitness to ...' certificates

NHS-related communications from
- Chief Medical Officer
- Department of Health
- Department for Work and Pensions
- NHS Executive
- Health authority/PCO
- National guidelines

Political information from
- British Medical Association
- General Practitioners Committee
- Local Medical Committee

Education and training
- Notifications of meetings
- Training updates/courses

Journals
- GP magazines
- Promotional and drug company

Other
- Questionnaires
- Research

Practice administration

Though you will need to complete sick notes for patients during the consultation, most other 'paperwork' should be done at other times. Forms need to be read, notes accessed and completed forms copied or scanned into the patient's records. The use of computerised medical records should help some form filling, but you will still often need the old paper notes, another reason for not starting form filling in your already too brief consultations.

This chapter covers issues relating to England, Wales and Scotland. Northern Ireland may have slight differences in forms and agencies to those discussed here.

THE GP POST BOX AND AN APPROACH TO PAPERWORK

Incoming mail should be opened by clerical staff, date-stamped and directed to the individual GP's in-tray. It may be scanned into the medical record before being passed to the GP.

Try to deal with your incoming mail daily to prevent a backlog. Set aside a weekly slot to catch up with the more time-consuming tasks such as long reports and document reading. Make use of surgery time when patients fail to turn up for quick tasks such as looking at individual pathology results. If you receive medical mail at home set aside a specific time to deal with it. Ideally you should handle, and deal with, each piece of paper only once.

Delegate if possible, direct items to other GPs if they know the patient better and expect them to do the same to you. Use administrative staff to fax, call patients and chase results and appointments. Contact the medical mailing lists, usually found at the back of the GP publications, to cancel subscriptions or send back unopened with 'return to sender' if you are inundated with unsolicited and unwelcome mail.

Some insurance and benefit forms come with a request that they be completed within a certain time.

Sign or initial everything you deal with, even if normal, and make clear any action undertaken in the patient's notes. Update patients' medical and prescribing records with significant results, new diagnoses, and drug changes instituted elsewhere. Some practices employ a staff member to upload the computer with relevant data you've highlighted on letters.

Box 12.2 Prioritising paperwork

- **Urgent** – do it now, certainly today
- **Soon** – this week
- **File** – future reference
- **Bin**

Make sure the practice has a system for a GP colleague to go through your post when you are away and find out who you are to cover in return.

Avoid building up a depressing 'journal mountain' (*Box 12.3*) Have a filing system for keeping information you may want to use later, particularly if you are taking the MRCGP exam in the future.

*See *Chapter 18: The MRCGP exam*.

Box 12.3   Keeping on top of the medical journals

- Identify and limit yourself to the few you really need to read*
- Stick to one GP magazine
- Limit yourself to one key article each week
- Aim not to let a new journal into the house/consulting room without processing the previous week's first!
- Use the online versions, e.g. *www.bmj.com*

SICKNESS CERTIFICATES

GPs are obliged to issue statutory certificates (*Box 12.4*) for patients unable to work due to ill health. Only a 'registered medical practitioner' can sign (*Box 12.5*) the official medical certificates, but the advice of other health professionals may need to be taken into account. Sick certificates can be used as evidence to support a claim for statutory sick pay for those in work and incapacity benefits for the unemployed. See *Box 12.6* for a detailed list of general practice forms.

Box 12.4   Which statutory certificate?

None	1–3 days illness
Self-certificate (SC1 or 2)	3–7 days illness
Med 3	After 7 days illness
	Open: no fixed return date
	Closed: return date stated within 14 days
Med 5	Backdated:
	– on basis of previous consultation, or
	– report from another doctor, e.g. discharge summary within last month
Med 4	Requested prior to Personal Capability Assessment (PCA)

Box 12.5   Completing certificates

- In ink
- Fully completed by doctor
- Issued once – duplicates for lost certificates must be completed by same doctor as original certificate and clearly state 'duplicate'
- Patient's name
- Date of examination
- Accurate diagnosis (otherwise see Med 6)
- Date of issue
- Address of doctor
- Doctor's signature

Adapted from *IB204: A Guide for Medical Practitioners*, Department of Work and Pensions, revised August 2004.

Clearly document in the patient's notes which certificate has been issued, the dates and illness details. Certificates are not infrequently lost and a duplicate may be requested. Fill out the details exactly as on the original but clearly mark as 'duplicate'. Advise patients to photocopy all certificates before passing them on to their employer or benefits office.

You must be honest and trustworthy when writing reports, completing or signing forms, or providing evidence in litigation or other formal enquiries. This means that you must take reasonable steps to verify any statement before you sign a document. You must not write or sign documents which are false or misleading because they omit relevant information. If you have agreed to prepare a report, complete or sign a document or provide evidence, you must do so without unreasonable delay.

Reproduced from 'Good Medical Practice', GMC.

Self-certificates

No statutory certificate is needed for absences of up to three working days. For absences between three and seven days patients should complete a self-certificate, SC1 for the unemployed and SC2 for employed patients, available from employers, the surgery or post offices. Employers should accept an SC2 and not expect GPs to issue certificates for short absences (see *Private sick certificates* below). Those on Job Seekers Allowance need an SC1 to confirm ill health and are then entitled to benefit without actively looking for work.

Med 3

A statement of incapacity to work, the Med 3 must be issued on the day of the consultation or within 24 hours. It can be 'open' with no specific return date for example 'four weeks', or 'closed' when a specific return to work date is agreed within the next 14 days. Within the first six months of illness a certificate can only be issued for up to six months. After this any time can be stipulated, even 'indefinite'.

You can include notes to the employer on a Med 3, e.g. recommending work changes or a gradual reintroduction to work.

Med 5

A special statement of incapacity to work, the Med 5 is issued under the following circumstances:

- Backdated, when a doctor agrees to issue a certificate based on their examination on a previous occasion to cover a period in the past. In these circumstances a Med 3 cannot be issued as over 24 hours have elapsed since the patient was seen. The doctor must be sure that they would have advised the patient to refrain from work for the entire period specified on the certificate. It can also be used to sign the patient off work for a future period of up to four weeks.
- On the basis of a report from another doctor, for example after an in-patient stay, when you are in receipt of the discharge summary. The report must not be more than one month old.

You *cannot* issue a Med 5 if you haven't seen the patient during the period of illness or have not received a report from another doctor who has seen the patient.

Med 4

A patient claiming incapacity benefit may be asked to attend a Personal Capability Assessment (PCA, see below). The PCA is usually applied after 28 weeks of incapacity but, depending on the medical condition, may be applied earlier. The patient will be sent a questionnaire to complete and asked to obtain a Med 4 from their doctor. The completion of the Med 4 overrides any previous Med 3 certificates and should be completed with particular care to include:

- main diagnosis causing incapacity
- any other illnesses
- effect of illness on function and ability to perform usual occupation
- treatment and prognosis
- ability of the patient to travel up to 90 minutes for PCA

Certain conditions will exempt a patient from attending for a PCA, for example tetraplegia and registered blindness, so careful completion of the Med 4 may help your patient avoid an unnecessary examination.

Med 6

Very rarely a doctor may judge it not to be in their patient's best interests to put a true or accurate diagnosis, for example cancer, on a Med 3, 4, or 5. In these circumstances a Med 6, found at the back of the Med 3 and Med 4 pads, should be completed and sent to the local benefits agency, their address can be found in the telephone directory. A fuller medical report may then be requested.

RM7

On the rare occasion you doubt a patient's incapacity but have issued a certificate and they are claiming state incapacity benefit you can request a PCA to be offered before 28 weeks. In such cases send an RM7, found at the back of the Med 3 pad, to the local Jobcentre Plus office.

DS1500

The DS1500 form should be completed for patients with a potentially terminal illness, who are likely to die within the next six months. This entitles them to 'special rules', enabling their claim for highest rate for Attendance Allowance (AA), Disability Living Allowance (DLA), or Incapacity Benefit (IB) to be processed without delay. Check they have already made a claim for these benefits. The forms are available from social security offices, Jobcentre Plus offices or downloadable from the DWP website. GPs may claim a fee for completing the DS1500 form.

Private sick notes

Patients may request certificates for less than seven days absence from work. The national guidelines of certification have been carefully negotiated and GPs are *not* usually obliged to issue any certificate for work absences of less than seven working days (the only rare exception is patients claiming state incapacity benefits who make repeated short-term claims). If a patient or employer insists on a certificate then a private sick certificate or note can be issued at your discretion and a fee can be charged.

Alternatively practices may produce a leaflet for patients to give to their employer explaining the rules of certification and that the employer can, with the patient's consent and for a fee, write to the GP to confirm the patient's attendance. This moves the administrative burden and cost of non-compliance with national guidance back to the employer rather than with GPs.

Difficulties arise where a patient requests a letter for an illness episode for which they have not consulted a doctor. Usually you should not issue a certificate but if you do issue then state that 'this patient *informs* me that they have been unwell' as you cannot actually confirm their illness.

Personal Capability Assessment

A person is asked to attend a PCA usually after a period of incapacity of 6 months. The level of assessment is based on the person's ability to perform certain day-to-day functions, and assesses whether they may be entitled to benefit without being expected to seek work.

Doctors approved by the DWP to ascertain a long-term claimant's fitness to do any sort of work, not necessarily their own job, undertake this clinical examination.

The GP who has been issuing the patient with sick notes is sent an IB113 form for completion before the PCA takes place, which requests detailed information on the patient's current illness, treatment and prognosis.

Once a PCA had been 'applied' or passed, and the patient deemed unfit for work, their GP will be informed in writing and further certificates will not be needed. If a patient appeals against the decision of a PCA, certificates will still be needed until the appeal is resolved.

Assessment for sick certification

GPs should work with patients with illness to both relieve symptoms and restore function, of which work may be an essential part. There are no absolute guidelines on amount of time off work required for specific conditions, as individuals vary in recovery times and psychological and social issues may prolong recovery. Good clinical care combined with consideration of occupational issues and rehabilitation may help prevent patients moving from short-term illness into a situation of long-term incapacity.

The common conditions responsible for most absence from work, e.g. depression and musculoskeletal problems, are often symptoms-based with little evidence of objective disease. Try to work thoughtfully with patients who request a prolonged absence from work which you feel may not be in their best interests. If you suspect depression is an underlying issue then address this. Conversely, persuading some patients that they need time off can be a problem, particularly if they are self-employed.

Hospital specialists should give advice and issue the certificates after an in-patient stay or operation.

Some patients will request time off work with a 'stress-related' or other non-specific condition, to allow them a period of recovery time when they are overwhelmed by stress or life crises, rather than illness. Try not to 'medicalise' social and personal problems; an alternative would be for the employer to consider compassionate leave rather than have the patient adopt the sick role.

Difficult situations arise when a patient requests a sickness certificate, yet you feel it inappropriate. Take time to explore the patient's agenda and to explain your reasons if you still consider it inappropriate. If you consider that problems at work may be a contributory factor, encourage the patient to discuss these with their employer. Sometimes you can negotiate and agree to a short certificate with a clear review date or return to work date. Discuss difficult cases with your colleagues or the GP the patient knows best.

WORKING WITH DISABILITY

In some circumstances you will need to write to employers in support of reduced duties for those who have been off work for serious illness or injury for sometime and are slowly integrating themselves back into work. These details can be included on a closed Med 3.

The Disability Discrimination Act (1995) requires employers to make reasonable adjustments to the work place for employees with long-term disability.

Disability Employment Advisors and Disability Service Teams, contactable through Job Centres, should provide individuals with advice and support on staying in employment, returning to work and starting work after a long absence.

As well as incapacity benefits there are also 'in work' benefits, making work a financially advantageous option for most people. The Working Tax Credit was introduced in 2003 and details should be available from employers or local Inland Revenue offices.

The New Deal for Disabled People (NDDP) helps those receiving disability or other health-related benefits find and retain work. Encourage patients to ask about this at their Job Centre.

OTHER FORMS AND CERTIFICATES

GP are asked to complete reports for a number of government agencies and organizations. These are not all a statutory requirement and may attract a fee*.

Particularly time-consuming are the Medical Attendant's Reports (MARs) for insurance and life assurance companies which require a full review of the patient's medical records.

*See *Chapter 1: Working in general practice* – Non-NHS income.

Find out which services generate a fee and get an idea of the rates for the commonly used services so you can advise patients before you agree to undertake a task. The practice should have a list of fees available at reception. Don't take the money yourself; direct the patient to the reception staff who will have a system for receiving money and issuing a receipt.

GP registrars should only be involved with completing forms that attract a fee if this fulfils an educational purpose.

> **Always ensure the patient has consented before releasing any medical information**
>
> **Don't agree to sign or complete forms or letters you don't fully understand**

Don't be pressurised into filling in forms or writing 'to whom it may concern' letters mid-surgery. Ask the patient to leave the matter with you and complete it after surgery so you can give it proper attention and have it copied into their notes. Give them a realistic timescale for its collection.

There may be an alternative to writing a 'to whom it may concern' letter. Housing departments often have specific forms to aid re-housing on medical grounds and will write to you for the information. Ask your colleagues for practice and local policies.

If it is not clear what information is required ask the patient or the third party to write down exactly what information they require.

You may need to refuse some requests. This will come with experience and confidence.

Attendance at the surgery

Patients should not need written confirmation that they have been to see a GP. Such requests are unreasonably using GPs to police the workforce and student population on behalf of employers and educational institutions. However, some practices may have a *pro forma*, e.g. 'This patient attended today' or you may agree to write a letter. Some doctors refuse to issue such 'certificates' and request that the patient asks their employer or college to write to them directly. The GP will then confirm attendance in writing. This offer is, unsurprisingly, rarely taken up.

Absence from school/college and sickness over exams

GPs are often asked to write certificates to cover a multitude of medical and non-medical situations for schools and colleges to explain short absences. Generally speaking the school should accept the word of a parent or student and not require a doctor's certificate.

Letters for illness during examination time, however, are usually justified as they may be acknowledged by examiners and affect a student's grades.

Schools may ask for reports on children with complex medical needs of which the school needs to be aware. Always ensure you have the patient's, or their parents' consent before sending these.

'Fitness to ...' certificates

Patients may request certificates, and examinations, confirming their fitness for a range of leisure and work activities. This is to absolve an organisation, such as a holiday tour operator, from responsibility should anything happen. However, the responsibility may then be passed back to you so beware.

Specific guidelines do exist on fitness to drive* and to fly as a passenger (see *Sources and further reading*) or when pregnant, when the woman should be advised to contact the airline directly. You may feel insufficiently knowledgeable to confirm fitness for some activities e.g. diving. Unless the organisation specifies the information it requires, or you know exactly what the activity involves and the level of fitness required, do not sign. Either refer the patient back to the organisation or issue a general, non-committal letter including phrases such as: 'To my knowledge this patient is currently fit and well' or 'This patient suffers from X and is being treated with Y'.

*See *Chapter 22: Clinical issues with legal stipulations* – Driving.

In some cases a full medical examination and completion of a certificate will be required, this will attract fee and the patient will need to book an appointment specifically for this.

Holiday cancellation

If a patient has cancelled a trip or holiday due to illness they may request a doctor's report to claim costs from their insurance company. You can only complete this if you saw the patient during their illness or have a report from another doctor who did. These types of report attract a fee.

Maternity certificates

Mat B1

Issued by a doctor or midwife within the last 20 weeks of confinement, i.e. at 20 weeks gestation, the Mat B1 allows women to claim Statutory Maternity Benefit (SMP) from their employer if employed or Maternity Allowance (MA) if self-employed or recently employed. Both are paid up to a maximum of 18 weeks, starting 11 weeks before the expected week of confinement at the earliest.

If a women is not entitled to SMP or MA, usually because not enough National Insurance has been paid, she may be treated as incapable of work from 6 weeks before expected delivery and 14 days after and issued a Med 3.

Sure Start Maternity Grant

Sure Start Maternity Grant (SSMG) is payable to low-income families to help with the costs of a new baby. Parents must have received advice from medical professional on maternal and child health care issues and have a signed form from a doctor or midwife to confirm this before making a claim.

BENEFITS

Millions of pounds each year are lost to patients in unclaimed benefits and as increased income from benefits. Few GPs have a full grasp of the complex and ever changing benefits and allowances for which their patients are eligible (*Box 12.7*). It's highly satisfying to advise a patient on a benefit to which they did not know they were entitled, as additional income can positively improve the health of individuals. Entitlement to some benefits depends on previous National Insurance contributions.

Box 12.6 General practice forms

DS1500	Fast access to maximum benefits for terminally ill patients likely to die within 6 months
D4	Application and medical report for Group 2 Driving licence
FP7 and FP8	Continuation cards for GP written notes
FP10	Standard prescription
FP10Comp	Standard prescription for computer use
FP10MDA	Prescription for prescribing in the treatment of addiction
FP92A	Application for medical exemption from prescription charges
FW8	Application for maternity exemption from prescription charges
GOS18	Request for ophthalmology opinion from optician to GP
HC2	Certificate for exemption from NHS charges
HSA1	Termination of pregnancy form
IB113	For completion before a PCA
MatB1	Form for claiming maternity benefits
Med 3–6	Statutory sickness certificates
RM7	Form to request a PCA where incapacity is in doubt
SC1 and 2	Self-certification forms

Box 12.7 Main state incapacity benefits and allowances

Benefit	Eligibility
Incapacity Benefit	<ul><li>payable if unable to work through illness or disability</li><li>Med 3 issued by GP until PCA applied</li><li>depends on NI contributions</li></ul>
Income Support and Disability Premium payable to a person unable to work because of incapacity	<ul><li>means-tested benefit for those whose lack of NI contributions means they are not eligible for incapacity benefit</li></ul>
Disability Living Allowance (DLA)	<ul><li>for those under 65, disabled and need either care or supervision or have reduced mobility</li><li>two components: mobility and care</li><li>higher and lower rates depend on level of disability and care needed.</li></ul>
Attendance Allowance (AA)	<ul><li>for over 65s needing care and/or supervision from another person</li></ul>

The DWP administers state benefits and produces a guide on completion of certificates *IB204, A Guide for Registered Medical Practitioners,* available via the DWP website. Be able to inform patients how to contact the local Citizens Advice Bureau and other local benefits advice agencies.

SOURCES AND FURTHER READING

1. DWP medical website, www.dwp.gov.uk/medical (gives access to accredited online training for issues relating to certification and fitness for work).
2. Information leaflets for patients available from Job Centres and Social Security offices:
   A guide to benefits
   Babies and children
   Sick or disabled
   Long term ill or disabled
   Ill or disabled because of work

3. Benefits Agency. *IB204: A Guide for Medical Practitioners.* Revised August 2004.
4. Hiscock J., Ritchie J. *The Role of GPs in Sickness Certification.* National Centre for Social Research on behalf of the DWP, 2001.
5. New Deal for Disabled People, www.newdeal.gov.uk/nddp
6. Sandell A. *Oxford Handbook of Patient's Welfare.* Oxford University Press, 1998.
7. Citizens Advice Bureau, www.citizensadvice.org.uk
8. Medical certificates and reports, *The new GMS and PMS contracts, Guidance for GPs,* General Practitioners Committee of the BMA, 2004.
9. The Cabinet Office. *'Making a Difference: Reducing GP Paperwork'* Her Majesty's Stationery Office, 2001.
10. Advising Patients about Air Travel, *Drug and Therapeutics Bulletin,* **34**: 30–32, 1996.
11. The Aviation Health Institute. *Contraindications to Air Travel: Guide for GPs,* www.aviation-health.org
12. British Thoracic Society. *Managing Passengers with Respiratory Disease: Planning Air Travel.* BTS, 2004.

Chapter 13
Extras in the working day

INTRODUCTION

In addition to clinical work GPs need to incorporate meetings, paperwork, telephone messages and the unexpected into their working day, all of which add stress if they are not anticipated. To maintain good medical practice, avoid errors and protect your sanity you need to develop your time management skills, your ability to delegate and learn to say no from time to time.

The new GP's share of these should be less than the partners so use this time to establish good habits.

DAY-TIME DUTY DOCTOR

Between 8 am and 6.30 pm weekdays each practice should have a duty doctor to deal with urgent calls and visits. New GPs should only be included in the duty doctor rota when they feel suitably confident, and GPRs should always be supervised.

The duty doctor will generally be responsible for:

- urgent visit requests
- urgent phone calls, prescription requests and abnormal results
- covering emergencies arising when the surgery doors are closed, e.g. lunchtime

Some practices reduce the duty doctor's routine work to allow for the on-call work as the unpredictability and longer working day can be stressful. Ensure you are well supported, delegate if possible and make time for meal and refreshment breaks. Leave your non-urgent paperwork until another day.

HIDDEN CONSULTATIONS

Patients increasingly communicate by letter, phone, fax and e-mail. Don't underestimate the work involved in these 'hidden consultations' as they may include requests for prescriptions, referrals, forms for completion or other action. Document all patient interactions in their medical record and only start a task when you have time to complete it.

If you can't deal with the problem without seeing the patient then ask the patient to make an appointment.

MANAGING INTERRUPTIONS

Interruptions are one of the more irksome parts of general practice whether during a surgery, paperwork session or coffee break. Although you are not at the end of a bleep, they can be harder to escape than in your hospital days.

If you feel you are having too many interruptions then discuss this with your colleagues. Staff may be using you as a 'soft touch' as you are the new person, and you may need to firm up your boundaries.

Reception staff should not interrupt your surgery unless absolutely urgent; medical emergencies and calls for truly urgent home visits are relatively rare. Try not to be pressurised into acting immediately with what a patient may consider is an emergency but you don't, e.g. needing a replacement Med 3 certificate, though be prepared to help out your battle-weary reception staff from time to time.

You may be happy (or not!) to be interrupted by calls from your nearest and dearest, so let reception staff know. Make clear the times when you absolutely cannot be disturbed and when you want to be disturbed, e.g. when expecting a call from a hospital consultant. Warn patients to expect an interruption if are waiting for a call, ask 'if they wouldn't mind waiting outside' to avoid breaking the confidentiality of the patient under discussion. Do oblige your professional colleagues, particularly nursing staff, who need a second opinion or a prescription mid-surgery.

THE TELEPHONE AND MESSAGES

> **Document all phone consultations in the medical record with date and time**

Make sure you know how to use the internal phone system.

Your practice should have a protocol for dealing with phone calls and messages left at reception from patients wishing to speak to a GP. Failure of such communication can lead to errors and complaints. There will usually be a message book, notes or e-mail directed to the relevant GP. Receptionists should ask the patient if they are able to deal with their request, e.g. to chase appointments, arrange transport, contact expected district nurses, before asking the patient to call back or taking a message. Requests for prescriptions should not be taken over the telephone.

Deal with your messages after each surgery, documenting all clinical contacts in the medical record with date and time.

Dealing with out of hours phone consultations is covered elsewhere*.

*See *Chapter 15: Out of hours work.*

Phoning patients back

Some GPs discourage patients leaving messages for them to phone them back. If you do reply to a request to phone a patient, treat this with the same respect as a face to face consultation – make sure you have the notes and you document the conversation in their records. Ask patients to make an appointment if they launch into a lengthy phone consultation for new problems.

Record failed attempts to return calls. Leave a neutral answerphone message if possible: 'This is Dr Y from the XX surgery returning your call at 12.30 pm on Tuesday 4th Jan. Please call again after 5.30 if you still need to speak to a doctor'. Try again later if you consider the problem might be serious from the tone of the message left for you.

If you have serious concerns and are persistently unable to get through, discuss this with a GP colleague. You may very occasionally need to consider a visit to ensure the patient is alright*.

*See *Chapter 14: Home visits –* If there is no answer.

Phone calls from concerned relatives

These can be difficult to manage, particularly the 'please don't tell them I called' and 'I want to know what's wrong with my father ...' varieties. You should actively seek the patient's consent and document this before discussing their care with a third party. Explain that you cannot discuss your patient's care, even to family members, without their consent[†]. If the patient does not want information to be disclosed you will have to pass this on to the enquirer. Alternatively, suggest the caller make an appointment to see you together with the patient.

†See *Chapter 21: Guidance for good professional practice –* Confidentiality.

MEETINGS

Although essential for management, service and educational aspects of working life (*Box 13.1*) meetings are often held at anti-social hours in order to fit into the overcrowded GP week. Ideally meetings should be well-planned, well-facilitated, kept to time and result in clear action plans to maximise productivity[‡].

‡See *Chapter 2: Working in the team.*

As a new member of the team it is important that you attend practice meetings as they should provide good insight into practice management and partner relations and you will be expected to contribute. You may not be invited to finance or partners' meetings.

GPRs should try to attend both a child protection case conference and a multidisciplinary mental health team meeting of a patient they know during the registrar year. Unfortunately these are often held at inconvenient times for GPs, such as mid-morning.

Keep a record of the educational meetings you attend for your personal development plan**.

**See *Chapter 20: Appraisal and revalidation.*

Box 13.1   GP meetings

Practice administration
- Practice meeting: day to day running of the practice
- Partners' meetings: overview of practice and inter-partner issues
- Finance meetings: review practice accounts with accountant
- Away days: meetings, for troubleshooting, team-building, forward planning

Clinical
- Multidisciplinary PCHT to discuss shared patients
- Case conferences
- Mental health review

Educational
- In-house meetings: hot topic review, audit, outside speaker to discuss services
- Journal club
- Postgraduate centre meetings
- Self-directed learning groups including MRCGP study groups and sessional or young practitioners' groups

Political/local planning
- PCO
- LMC

Chapter 14
Home visits

INTRODUCTION

Home visits continue to form an important part of UK general practice both for routine and emergency care. Consultations with patients in their own home can yield valuable information; you are more likely to make an appropriate OT or social services referral following a visit than a short surgery consultation. Although it is a privilege to be welcomed into people's homes, visits can be time-consuming, navigation and parking frustrating and home may not provide an ideal setting for a full clinical assessment.

This chapter concentrates on visits during the working day, which tend to be for planned review of housebound patient or patients too ill to come to the surgery. Out of hours visits are dealt with in *Chapter 15: Out of hours work.*

PRACTICAL PREPARATIONS

*See *Chapter 13: Extras in the working day* – Day-time duty doctor.

Find out how you will be contacted on duty doctor or on call days*. Make sure the practice staff and OOH service have your mobile telephone number and that is it charged and switched on. Do GPs in your practice carry a bleep as well? If so make sure you know how to use it.

You are required to have transport for visiting. Have little to identify your vehicle as a doctor's to reduce break-ins and check with your practice manager for local doctors' parking regulations. If your vehicle is off the road and you cannot get a replacement negotiate with your colleagues to undertake visits that can be done on foot.

†See *Chapter 6: Practical preparations for clinical work* – Your bag.

You will need a fully equipped doctor's bag†.

SAFETY PRECAUTIONS

Most visits during the day raise few safety risks. The patients are usually elderly, housebound and well known to the practice. In the rare scenario that

---

Box 14.1   Visiting: safety precautions

- Always inform someone of the destination and expected duration of any visit you undertake unaccompanied
- Carry limited quantities of drugs and prescriptions
- Lock your car and your bag if left in the car
- Consider carrying a personal alarm
- Ask a family member to come out and meet you on unfamiliar estates
- Ask the police to meet you at the address if violence is a possibility

---

you have concerns from the patient's medical records or the tone of the visit request, try to get as much information as possible before visiting. Trust your instincts and perhaps ask one of your colleagues to go with you (see *Box 14.1*).

VISITS DURING THE WORKING DAY

Visits are usually scheduled visits to housebound patients needing review or to nursing or residential homes, or visits requested for or by patients too unwell to come to the surgery. Requests may also come from PHCT staff, particularly district nurses.

Reception staff should have a system to document visit requests from patients and carers with the reason for the request.

Most GPs visit at lunchtime so requests should be made in the morning by a stipulated time. Requests at other times will usually be passed to the duty doctor. It is rare for a GP to need to leave mid-surgery for an emergency visit.

Apart from the housebound, patients should be encouraged to attend the surgery if at all possible.

Joint visits with nurses or specialists such as psychiatrists, psychogeriatricians and the palliative care team can be particularly useful but take some planning.

Visits are usually distributed evenly among the visiting GPs for that day or allocated to the duty doctor or GP who knows the patient best. As a new GP you may cover absent partners' patients. There will be days when you need to limit the number of visits you can undertake due to other commitments, e.g. meetings and exams. Let your colleagues and reception staff know when this is the case.

AN APPROACH TO VISITING

GPRs should visit with their trainer for the first few weeks before visiting alone. As with all consultations, GPRs should be supervised at all times by a named GP available by phone.

Always inform reception and a GP colleague if you need to leave for a visit mid-surgery or will be delayed back for your surgery. They can appease, and perhaps see, some of your waiting patients.

Before you go

It is helpful to telephone the patient before visiting to find out the exact problem and whether you need any specific additional equipment, e.g. a nebuliser. Confirm the address and ask for directions. With experience you may be able to negotiate an alternative to a visit such as:

- attendance at the surgery
- telephone advice
- a prescription
- referral to another health professional, e.g. district nurse for a dressing problem

If possible, speak to the patient's usual GP or other member of the PHCT who knows the patient.

Ensure you have the medical records or a comprehensive computer summary together with an updated medication list. Let reception know where you are going and that you are effectively unavailable unless you are on call.

While you're there

Once you've found the place and introduced yourself, deal with the consultation much as you would in surgery. Be vigilant in keeping pets and children's fingers out of your bag. Ask to have the TV and distracting music turned off so you can concentrate on the consultation. Ensure you have good light and the patient in the best setting for a full examination, which may mean moving to another room. If you are unsure how to manage the patient you can always return to the surgery and seek advice from a colleague and call the patient back with a management plan.

Write brief notes on site and leave prescriptions, investigation and referral paperwork with the patient. Update the computer record when you get back. Some practices have the luxury of laptops linked to the surgery system so notes can be accessed and written up at the patient's home.

If there is no answer

Check you have the correct address, shout through the letterbox, or look through a window and telephone from your mobile before assuming the worst, only to find they've gone to the hairdresser! If there is no response and you have a high index of concern, based either on previous history or the reason for the visit request, consider calling your local A&E and the ambulance service to check if they are currently dealing with the patient. Only then consider calling the police to help you with access. Breaking the door down is rarely necessary. If you are less concerned then consider leaving a note, and telephone the patient later.

On your return

Complete the computer and prescribing records. Replace any drugs or dressings dispensed from your bag. Arrange any investigations and referrals, including to PHCT members. Log any plans for future visits or telephone reviews and make sure these are adhered to.

SPECIAL CASES

Terminally ill patients

Patients with terminal illness can usually visit the surgery early in the illness, but become housebound as their illness progresses. Looking after a patient through a terminal illness is often a distressing but rewarding aspect of general practice. Registrars should try to get involved in the care of such a patient. A weekly, or fortnightly, visit with the same doctor can be very reassuring to patients and their family. Always leave a good half an hour for such visits, have a cup of tea, and don't feel a need to 'do' anything beyond symptom control, reassurance and acting as liaison between hospital, nursing and palliative care staff. A visit to bereaved relatives after a death is usually greatly appreciated.

Elderly housebound patients

Aside from dealing with the presenting complaint, use the visit for a general review including any long term illness review, medication check and removal of obsolete medicines (with the patient's permission), give a flu jab, and offer health promotion advice. Check the patient has adequate support, identify any safety issues e.g. loose carpets, need for bath rails, and with the patient's agreement make any necessary referrals to social services or OT.

The acutely mentally ill patient

Even when a crisis is brewing and a mental health section possible, you may still be able to persuade a patient to come to the surgery for assessment, perhaps accompanied by their CPN. You may feel more secure at the surgery and have help and advice more readily to hand.

Registrars should accompany their trainer on a section visit before undertaking a section themself. Sectioning patients is covered in depth in *Chapter 22: Clinical issues with legal stipulations* – The Mental Health Act and the acutely mentally ill patient.

Chapter 15
Out of hours work

INTRODUCTION

Out of hours (OOH) covers 6.30 pm to 8 am weekdays and all day at weekends and bank holidays. Practices will have their own system for covering emergencies during the day*.

*See *Chapter 13 Extras in the working day* – Day-time duty doctor.

Your practice telephone system should have a message when the practice is closed explaining how, in the case of emergencies, patients can contact the OOH provider or connect patients directly.

Over the last 20 years OOH work has become increasingly unpopular amongst GPs and shown to contribute disproportionately to feelings of stress, fatigue and fear of violence. The nGMS contract gives practices the option to opt out of the OOH commitment for their patients and to hand the responsibility for this to the PCO. The vast majority of UK practices have chosen this opt out and have their global sum reduced to reflect this[†].

†See *Chapter 1: Working in general practice.*

GPs are still core workers in any OOH service and all new GPs must be able to show they have achieved some core competencies (see later) before embarking on unsupervised OOH work.

‡See *Chapter 3: Working in the wider health service* – NHS Direct.

The role of NHS Direct[‡] is expanding as part of an integrated OOH service incorporating GP services, walk-in centres, pharmacies, A&E, ambulance and community nursing teams.

Some organisations have chosen to use the term 'unscheduled primary care' as an alternative to OOH. This reflects a shift from seeing emergencies to seeing patients whose personal preference is to see a GP in evenings and weekends. Some GPs have concerns about the potential fragmentation of services that may result from this.

PROVISION OF OUT OF HOURS CARE

Although OOH providers can still be the individual practice, it is more likely to be a PCO-run or commissioned service, using multidisciplinary team models of care.

Many of the current OOH systems are based on the old cooperatives. GPs and other health care workers are contracted to work a shift system. The service provides OOH care using a combination of telephone consultations, face to face contacts at a primary care centre and home visits. Increasingly nurses are the first line of contact, or triage, for these services, and from 2006 it is planned that NHS Direct will be the single point of access for all OOH contacts.

PCOs may provide and manage more 'innovative' models, combining the services of A&E and walk-in centres with primary care services.

Although GP practices may have chosen to opt out of OOH work, individual GPs may do OOH sessions for which they are paid a fee.

PCOs may commission OOH work from other providers, most notably deputising services. Introduced in the 1960's, these profit-making organisations employ doctors to do OOH sessions and hold contracts with some PCOs to provide the primary care OOH service for their area.

All OOH providers are expected to reach certain competencies and are inspected annually*.

*See *Chapter 3: Working in the wider health service* – Healthcare Commission.

OUT OF HOURS AND THE GP REGISTRAR

> **GPRs must always be adequately supervised when doing any out of hours work**

OOH work still forms a core part of UK general practice and all GPRs' training must include time spent in an OOH setting. Accreditation is dependent on GPRs demonstrating that they have achieved the five core competencies required (see *Box 15.1*). A significant proportion of the GPRs pay is in the form of an OOH allowance.

When a PCO has set up or commissioned an OOH provider, they must ensure there is provision for training and supervision of GPRs.

The number of OOH sessions a GPR should undertake is not set in stone but the Committee of General Practice Education Directors (COGPED) recommends 12, of about 6 hours duration, during the year. These sessions must be supervised by a GP trainer, either the registrar's own trainer or a different trainer, or another clinical supervisor who does not necessarily have to be a GP but will have had training for this role. If your trainer is not undertaking your OOH supervision they must be satisfied that your clinical supervisor is competent. Your trainer or supervisor should supervise both the care you provide to patients and your learning experience. GPRs must feel satisfied that they are receiving adequate supervision OOH and should discuss this with their trainer or VTS course organiser if not.

GPRs must keep documented evidence of their achieved OOH competencies and experience. This should include self-assessment and reflection

---

Box 15.1   Core competencies for OOH work

1. The ability to deal with medical emergencies
2. The ability to use the 'system' OOH e.g. admitting patients at weekends, understanding availability of support services
3. An understanding of the organisational aspects of NHS OOH care e.g. different methods of delivery
4. Effective communication skills for OOH care
5. Self-care in OOH work, e.g. time and stress management

---

and any formal or informal assessments or comments from supervisors and other colleagues. OOH logbooks are available for this.

*See *Chapter 5: Contract and finances.*
†See *Chapter 16: Educational aspects of the GP registrar year.*

OOH work commitments should be included in the GPR contract* and educational contract†.

If you work a night shift you should have the following day off.

The Deanery and trainers should ensure that registrars are not working beyond the European Working Times Directive, which came into place in August 2004.

CONSULTING OUT OF HOURS

Always take a thorough history of the presenting problem and ask specifically about:

- **concurrent medical conditions**
- **past medical history**
- **current medication**
- **allergies**

Document all consultations with time and date.

The vast majority of patients use OOH services appropriately for medical emergencies that cannot wait until their own surgery is next open. Most calls will be from parents with young children, the elderly or their carers. There are many reasons for people to call: having responsibility for someone else, a previous missed diagnosis, fear about a specific illness, such as meningitis, or failure of self-treatment. Understanding people's fears may help you reassure the caller and perhaps reduce your own exasperation at what you may otherwise consider a waste of time.

Decision-making in emergency consultations

Use the algorithm in *Box 15.2* for all GP emergency contacts, in or out of hours‡.

‡See also *Chapter 10: Referrals* – Emergency referrals.

An approach to out of hours telephone consultations

Most OOH consultations start with a telephone call. Introduce yourself, try and speak to the patient directly if possible. Use a general opener such as 'What can I do for you?' even if you have some patient details, and allow the patient to talk before you ask direct questions. Management decisions may be informed by how well, breathless or anxious the patient sounds. If you cannot make a reasonable assessment over the telephone then a face to face contact,

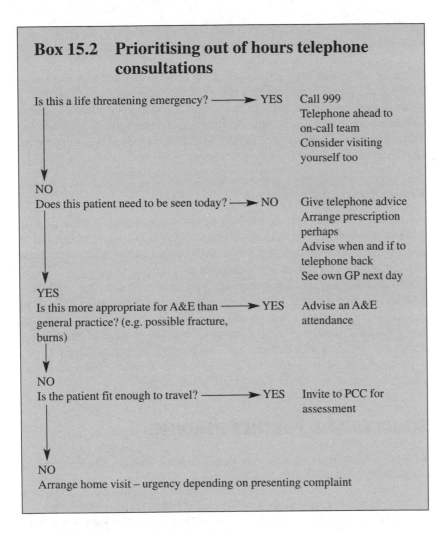

Box 15.2   Prioritising out of hours telephone consultations

Is this a life threatening emergency? ⟶ YES → Call 999
Telephone ahead to on-call team
Consider visiting yourself too

NO

Does this patient need to be seen today? ⟶ NO → Give telephone advice
Arrange prescription perhaps
Advise when and if to telephone back
See own GP next day

YES

Is this more appropriate for A&E than general practice? (e.g. possible fracture, burns) ⟶ YES → Advise an A&E attendance

NO

Is the patient fit enough to travel? ⟶ YES → Invite to PCC for assessment

NO

Arrange home visit – urgency depending on presenting complaint

visit or invitation to the PCC is essential. Those with poor English, learning difficulties, high anxiety or under the influence of drugs or alcohol can be particularly difficult to assess over the telephone.

If a patient calls a second time after initial advice then have a low threshold for a face to face contact. Let patients know if there will be a long wait for visits and request they call back should they deteriorate. They may decide that they can make their way to you at the PCC.

Negotiating visits

Experienced GPs will try to discourage requests for home visits when they are not clearly indicated. Patients will usually be seen quicker if they attend the primary care centre and it is a more efficient use of a health professional's time. As a new GP you should not be solely responsible for declining visit requests. Negotiating this takes practice. Observe how other GPs do this: it is a useful skill to learn: 'I think we should see you. Would you like to come in to ....? Generally you will not have to wait long.'

If a patient insists on a visit that you deem unnecessary and a confrontation seems likely, then you may need to agree and save yourself stress. You should make it clear on the feedback to the patient's GP that the patient insisted. Children with fevers *can* go out, despite what parents believe, however, the 'lack of transport' plea can be difficult to get round unless you work for an OOH provider that arranges patient transport.

Prescribing out of hours

Most OOH providers provide medical equipment and drugs. Check exactly what is provided and make suggestions if you think something vital is missing. Some GPs prefer to take their own medical bag with equipment and medication so they know exactly what they are carrying.

Avoid giving injections for chronic or recurrent self-limiting conditions such as migraine or irritable bowel syndrome as this may encourage patient expectation of a repeat in the future. Buccal and rectal alternatives are usually available. Don't hesitate to use injections for severe chest pain, renal colic, intractable vomiting with dehydration, etc., pending transfer to hospital.

*See Chapter 8: Prescribing – Prescribing over the telephone.

Prescriptions can be telephoned through to local chemists*, but ensure that you have 'safety-netted' particularly well if you do this.

SOURCES AND FURTHER READING

1. Hallam L. Primary medical care outside normal working hours: review of published work. *BMJ*, **308**: 249–253, 1994.
2. Hopton J., Hogg R., McKee I. Patients' accounts of calling the doctor out of hours: qualitative study in one general practice. *BMJ*, **3131**: 991–994, 1996.
3. COGPED. *Out of Hours (OOH) Training for GP Registrars*. Position paper. April 2004.
4. London Deanery Trainer's Guide. *Out of Hours Experience of GP Registrars*. December 2003.
5. NHS Direct, www.nhsdirect.nhs.uk

Chapter 16
Educational aspects of the GP registrar year

INTRODUCTION

The 12 months as a registrar pass quickly and you are unlikely to fit in all that you wish to. You may catch up with some of the elements you couldn't fit in, including the MRCGP exam after the registrar year. Learning and training continues throughout your career; bear this in mind before you start to feel overwhelmed by how much there is to know.

Remember the bottom line aims for the year are:

1. **To conduct a surgery safely, efficiently and confidently**
2. **Successful completion of summative assessment and acquisition of your certificate of training (JCPTGP or PMETB)***

*See *Chapter 17: Summative assessment* – Administration.

SUMMATIVE ASSESSMENT AND THE MRCGP EXAM

Summative assessment is often described as a test of minimum competence. Successful completion of all four modules is a requirement of GP training. The MRCGP exam is deemed an exam of excellence and can be taken during or after the registrar year.

Chapters 17 to 19 are devoted to these assessments. In your first few months, start *thinking* about summative assessment and the MRCGP exam and plan your educational timetable for the year with these in mind. Refer to the latest exam regulations and note all deadlines for applications and submissions as well as the dates of exams (See *Sources and further reading*).

THE BASICS

Adult learning

General practice training places a lot of emphasis on 'adult learning' i.e. self-directed, experiential and adapted to your personal needs. Your trainer, course organisers and fellow adult learners, e.g. VTS or study group, should work with you on this.

All registrars will have had different experiences before joining general practice and will therefore have different learning needs. You need to create a Personal Development Plan (PDP) which will highlight your aims for the year, direct your study and become a record of your learning. It will also contribute to your appraisal documentation[†].

†See *Chapter 20: Appraisal and revalidation*.

Making the most of your trainer

Trainers have many roles: they are your tutor, colleague, mentor, role model, counsellor, referee, as well as employer. As a result the registrar–trainer relationship can be quite intense and probably unlike any other in your medical training.

Learn how best to use them and when to ask for help. You may find other partners in the practice have expertise in certain areas and you can direct some of your queries to them. Where possible, store up queries for your weekly tutorial.

Plan your tutorials together and review the topics list as you progress through the year. Remember that you must be supervised whenever you are working so reinforce this point if you feel 'neglected'.

Most registrars get on well with their trainers, although problems do occasionally arise. Try to discuss any issues directly with your trainer, but your course organiser should be approached if you would find this too difficult or if a problem remains unresolved. If you feel this is not possible or it fails to produce results then approach the Associate Dean (or Associate Director) at your local deanery. Your regional BMA office may be able to help BMA members, especially for contractual and employment difficulties*.

*See *Chapter 5: Contract and finances* – Difficulties arising with your contract.

Educational contract

This contract can supplement your employment contract and may be drawn up with your trainer. It should define the aims and objectives of your year, specify time for tutorials and study leave and provide a framework for planning your induction period, tutorials and assessments. Many of the VTS schemes produce a locally approved contract.

Deanery information

At the start of your registrar year your local deanery may send you a lot of information about the deanery and summative assessment. However, most deanery websites contain this information and have further useful details about training. Information on summative assessment and the MRCGP exam can be obtained from the relevant websites (see *Sources and further reading*).

Study leave

This is covered in Chapter 5 (*Contract and finances* – Study leave). You are entitled to a minimum 30 days study leave. You should also be entitled to an education support allowance from your deanery. Find out how to make an application for reimbursement early in the year. You will normally have to apply prior to attending an educational event and have the approval of your trainer and the deanery so plan well ahead.

MAKING THE MOST OF THE EDUCATIONAL OPPORTUNITIES

There are many opportunities for learning in different contexts (*Box 16.1*). Ensure you have protected time and a structure for reflecting on what you've learnt. Make the most of your study leave entitlement and claim financial reimbursement from the deanery up to your maximum allowance. The registrar induction period can be usefully spent sitting in with members of the PHCT and meeting other providers of health care. However, you can arrange to do this at any time in your year if you think these opportunities fulfil a learning need.

Box 16.1 Educational opportunities in the year

Surgery-based
- Surgeries
- Weekly tutorials with trainer or other partner
- Sitting in with and accompanying trainer or other partners and PHCT members
- Joint surgeries
- Practice meetings
- Complaints and Significant Event Analyses

Out of the surgery
- Visits – both with other GPs and by yourself
- Out of hours work*
- VTS half-day release course
- VTS residential
- Specialist outpatients
- Local practice visits (arrange via other registrars or via the VTS)
- Practice swap with contrasting training practice
- Postgraduate centre academic meetings
- Courses

Community-based health services[†]
It may be possible to arrange to spend time with:
- district nurses
- community midwives
- health visitors
- community mental health team
- community palliative care team
- community drug and alcohol services
- intermediate care team
- family planning clinic
- community-based sexual health clinic
- pharmacist
- optician
- podiatrist
- funeral director

*See *Chapter 15: Out of hours work.*

†See *Chapter 2: Working in the team.*

Weekly tutorials

Devise a flexible programme of relevant topics with your trainer. Ensure variety so include:

- clinical topics
- practice management
- management of difficult patients
- reviewing your videos
- discussion of ethical, political and service issues

Ideally both you and your trainer should spend time preparing for each tutorial to maximise the benefits to you. Your trainer should arrange for another partner to teach you if they are away. Other partners may be better suited to giving a tutorial on a subject of their particular expertise.

Organise regular 3-monthly reviews with your trainer to reassess your learning needs and to evaluate the preceding months.

Get your trainer to fill in the structured trainer's report as you progress through the year*.

*See *Chapter 17: Summative assessment* – The structured trainer's report.

VTS educational course

Vocational Training Schemes organise an ongoing educational programme during term time that registrars should attend as part of their working week. This is normally organised as a weekly half-day release scheme although some VTSs may opt for a whole day every fortnight. Formats vary but these sessions may include presentations often with outside speakers, small group work and informal discussion (*see Box 16.2*).

Although the programme is usually constructed by the course organisers, input from the participants is actively encouraged so try to make sure topics that are of relevance to you are included.

The VTS is an excellent source of information and support. It is a forum to discuss problems, find out more about local courses, get advice about exams and discuss future plans. Once you have found your feet in the year, you may find it useful to set up a study group with a small group of people from the VTS with similar aims, e.g. passing the MRCGP exam or ongoing self-directed learning.

VTS residential course

These courses are normally a few days long and are organised by most VTS. They are often set in pleasant surroundings away from your local area. As well as focusing on an educational topic, they give you a chance to get to know your colleagues from the VTS better. Expect these to occur at least once in your registrar year.

Box 16.2 Possible topics for VTS half-day release course

Practical sessions
- CPR training and certification session (compulsory for the MRCGP exam)
- Consultation skills, e.g reviewing videos, role-playing with actors
- Self-defence

Clinical topics
- Specialty update
- Unfamiliar clinical topics, e.g. substance abuse, complementary medicine, domestic violence

Non-clinical topics
- Communication skills
- Continuing medical education, e.g. personal development plans
- Critical appraisal
- People and time management
- Financial and business management
- Stress management
- Careers in general practice
- The doctor–patient relationship, e.g. small group work focusing on a problem patient

Visits
- Local practices
- Local hospice
- PCO/ Health Authority
- RCGP
- Local prison
- Walk in centre

Specialist hospital outpatients

Many consultants and nurse specialists are happy for you to sit in with them. Contact local specialists in clinical areas in which you want more training. You may feel like a medical student again but get the most out of the experience by discussing problem cases and referrals to the specialist.

Practice swap

Get a taste of another type of practice. Ideally swap for a week with a registrar or working in a different area or practice. Doing locums following your training provides similar experience.

National Conference for GPs to Be

This conference was first held in 2004 and is likely to become an annual event. It is organised jointly by the RCGP and GP Registrars Subcommittee of the GPC*.

*See *Chapter 3: Working in the wider health service.*

Courses

Look at your deanery website, the *BMJ* or *BJGP* for information on courses that interest you. Ask your trainer to keep you informed of local courses and the VTS may provide you with some details.

Other opportunities

You can get involved in politics, e.g. representing GPRs on the Registrars' Subcommittee of the GPC or your local deanery registrars committee. You may be able to sit on the panel at interviews for prospective registrars. Additional leave should be granted for these activities.

Sources for individual study

Individual study of course remains an important part of learning (*Box 16.3*).

USEFUL QUALIFICATIONS AND SKILLS

Some skills and qualifications (*Box 16.4*) will allow you to pursue an interest, broaden your scope for generating income for your future practice, and make you more employable. Approved regional courses are available for many of the practical skills. Select areas where you lack confidence as well as subjects that interest you.

The diploma exams

There are many postgraduate qualifications that are relevant to general practice. *Box 16.5* lists some of those that are most commonly undertaken by GPs and prospective GPs. These optional assessments 'recognise an interest' in a specialty and are useful to consolidate experience acquired in your SHO jobs. They may be best undertaken towards the end of or after a specialty attachment. Some require you to have a minimum 6 months experience in a specialty. They may be difficult to fit into the overcrowded registrar year.

Contact the individual Royal Colleges / Faculties for details and application.

Box 16.3   Sources for individual study

Textbooks
- See *Sources and further reading* at the end of each chapter

GP press*
- *Pulse, Doctor, GP, The Practictioner, Update, Med Economics*
- You will be overwhelmed if you read them all. One a week may be best

Journals
- *British Medical Journal (BMJ), British Journal of General Practice (BJGP), Drugs and Therapeutics Bulletin* (DTB)*

Guidelines
- NICE guidance should be sent to you. You can subscribe to an monthly e-newsletter via the website, www.nice.org.uk
- There are lots of other sources of guidelines (See *Appendix 1: Useful websites*). Ask your trainer and colleagues

CPD modules
- Interactive modules on various clinical and non-clinical topics are available on the web including: **BMJ Learning**, www.bmjlearning.com, **doctors.net** www.doctors.net.uk (see also *Appendix 1: Useful websites*)

Phased Evaluation Programme (PEP)
- CD-ROM available from RCGP
- Self assessment tool covering clinical and non-clinical topics relevant to general practice

Chief Medical Officer (CMO) updates/ letters*
- You should automatically receive these
- Highlight important policy changes and DOH priorities

* The Medical Mailing Company holds a database on to which you can register to receive or cancel these publications. Freephone 0800 626 387.

Box 16.4   Qualifications and skills for the GP registrar

Qualifications and practical skills
- MRCGP
- Cardiopulmonary resuscitation (compulsory for MRCGP exam)
- IUCD insertion and subdermal contraceptive implant insertion
- Minor surgery
- Diploma exams, e.g. Family Planning, Child Health, DRCOG, and Geriatric Medicine
- RCGP certificate in the management of drug misuse

Box 16.5   Diploma examinations

- Diploma of the Royal College of Obstetricians and Gynaecologists (DRCOG), Royal College of Obstetricians and Gynaecologists, www.rcog.org.uk
- Diploma in Child Health (DCH), The Royal College of Paediatrics and Child Health, www.rcpch.ac.uk
- Diploma of the Faculty of Family Planning (DFFP), Faculty of Family Planning and Reproductive Health Care, www.ffprhc.org.uk
  Also provide information on IUCD and subdermal contraceptive implant insertion
- Diploma in Geriatric Medicine (DGM), The Royal College of Physicians, www.rcplondon.ac.uk

SOURCES AND FURTHER READING

1. National Office for Summative Assessment, www.nosa.org.uk
2. Royal College of General Practitioners, www.rcgp.org.uk
3. List of deaneries with contacts details, www.copmed.org.uk/Deaneries
4. Swanick T., Chana N. *The Study Guide for General Practice Training.* Radcliffe Medical Press, 2003.
5. Warren E. *Tutorials for the General Practice Registrar.* Butterworth-Heinemann, 2002.
6. Rosenthal J. *et al. The Successful GP Registrar's Companion.* Churchill Livingstone, 2003.
7. Hall M., Dwyer D., Lewis T. *The GP Training Handbook, 3rd edition.* Blackwell Science, 1999.

8. Birtwistle J. *et al.* *Oxford Handbook of General Pratice.* Oxford University Press, 2002.
9. Knot A., Polmear A. *Practical General Practice, 4th Edition.* Butterworth-Heinemann, 2003.
10. Cartwright S., Godlee C. *Churchill's Pocketbook. General Practice, 2nd Edition.* Churchill Livingstone, 2003.

Chapter 17
Summative assessment

INTRODUCTION

Summative assessment (SA) aims to ensure basic competence in all new GPs. Successful completion of all the four components is a pre-requisite for your qualification as a GP in the UK (*Box 17.1*).

Intended as a comprehensive assessment, it tests medical knowledge (and an ability to apply it), clinical skills, communication skills (written and oral), as well as an ability to critically analyse your own working practices.

Most GPRs should have no problem in passing this assessment. Only about 4% of registrars ultimately fail and further training is usually arranged for this group. In many cases components can be re-sat or resubmitted following input from your trainer, course organiser and deanery.

Despite assurances given in the official documentation the components do involve a lot of work, but it should not take over your life. You should have protected time for the written work and support should be forthcoming from your trainer and VTS colleagues.

Box 17.1   Summative assessment components

1. **MCQ**
   - COGPED MCQ, or
   - MRCGP MCQ paper
2. **Assessment of consultation skills**
   - COGPED video, or
   - MRCGP video (MRCGP/SA single route), or
   - Simulated surgery
3. **Written submission of practical work**
   - COGPED audit, or
   - Project marked under the National Project Marking Schedule
4. **Structured trainer's report**

ADMINISTRATION

Familiarise yourself with the latest national guidelines available on the website of the National Office for Summative Assessment (NOSA). Application forms for summative assessment are downloadable from this site and should be filled in and sent to your local deanery.

Each deanery has a Summative Assessment Office which may provide further local information on summative assessment. This office also administers the Committee of General Practice Education Directors (COGPED) components and arranges the signing of your VTR1 form on successful completion of your summative assessment at the end of the registrar year. This form is returned to you and you will then need to send it to the Joint Committee on Postgraduate Training for General Practice (JCPTGP). You will also have to send the JCPTGP your VTR2 forms which confirm completion of hospital posts. Once all the completed forms have been received, the JCPTGP will issue a certificate which enables you to practice in the UK.

At the time of writing the JCPTGP is being replaced by the Postgraduate Medical Education and Training Board (PMETB) so update yourself by checking their websites*. All GPRs should have received a national training number and this should be entered on all submissions and correspondence.

*See *Sources and further reading* and *Chapter 3: Working in the wider health service*.

The RCGP provides further information on taking one or more modules of the membership exam as part of summative assessment[†].

†See *Chapter 18: The MRCGP exam*.

Your practice should provide all the equipment you need to undertake summative assessment and it should not cost you anything if you undertake the COGPED components.

DEADLINES

You will need to structure your educational year around the exam dates and submission deadlines (*Box 17.2*) which you should have on your year planner[‡].

‡See also *Chapter 16: Educational aspects of the GP registrar year*.

Box 17.2 Summative assessment year planner

Month

1	Familiarise yourself with summative assessment guidance from your deanery and the NOSA. Check application deadlines and confirm examination dates. Read through the trainer's report; fill in as you progress. Fill in application form for summative assessment
2 and 3	Start considering written work topic Start videos for practice and improving consultation skills
4	First chance to sit summative assessment MCQ
5	Check the application dates for simulated surgery (if undertaking this)
6	
7	Submit video or sit simulated surgery from now on
8	
9	Deadline for submission of written work and video (end of month)
10	
11	Submit trainer's report by end of month
12	Get VTR1 form completed by trainer and deanery Apply for JCPTGP/PMETB certificate

---

THE COMPONENTS

The basic four components of summative assessment are set by the COGPED. As the assessment has evolved more options have become available, with some overlap with the MRCGP exam.

You may need the permission of your local deanery office to ensure funding for any non-COGPED components and you will have to pay for any MRCGP components you opt for.

You also need to inform your deanery office of your chosen method for each component; bear in mind that once you have chosen a method, this cannot be changed. You will therefore also have to decide early on in your registrar year whether or not to apply for the MRCGP exam.

MCQ paper

The COGPED MCQ is a 3-hour paper. It is held four times a year in each region. It can be taken after 3 months experience as a GPR. The NOSA discourages any earlier attempts. The pass rate is currently 94%.

The topics covered are :

- **Internal medicine** – medicine, therapeutics, surgical diagnosis, psychiatry, geriatrics – 45% of total
- **Child health** – one sixth of total
- **Womens'/mens' health** - one sixth of total
- **External medicine** – ENT, eyes, dermatology – one sixth of total
- **Practice management** – 5% of total

The paper consists of:

- 170 items of standard true/false questions
- 80 extended matching item questions
- 10 single best answer style questions

Examples of these questions are included in *Box 17.3*.

The paper is not negatively marked, so make sure you answer all the questions.

Alternatively you can sit the MRCGP MCQ paper, held twice a year. Your deanery office will need written evidence from the RCGP of your success in this to complete your VTR1 form.

There should be no need to revise specific topics for the COGPED MCQ. However, the MRCGP exam syllabus* may be a useful guide to relevant topics. In addition, the RCGP has produced Phased Evaluation Program (PEP) self assessment CD-ROMs which cover many aspects of general practice and will give you practice in answering MCQ-style questions.

*See *Chapter 18: The MRCGP exam.*

Consultation skills

You can either submit a video or undertake the simulated surgery currently organised by the Leicester, Northamptonshire and Rutland (LNR) Deanery.

Box 17.3   Examples of MCQs

Standard multiple choice question
An umbilical hernia in a 6-month-old child requires:
    A urgent surgical repair
    B surgical repair at the age of 12 months
    C reassurance of the parent
    D none of the above

Extended matching item question
Select the single most appropriate diagnosis for each of these case histories. A diagnosis may appear once, more than once or not at all:
    A conjunctivitis
    B anterior uvetitis
    C acute (closed angle) glaucoma
    D subconjunctival haemorrhage
    E vitreous haemorrhage
    F retinal detachment
1. A 35-year-old man who is short-sighted presents to you describing a loss of vision in one eye. He describes it as a 'curtain coming down' across one eye.
2. A 23-year-old woman presents with bilateral red eyes. She describes symptoms of itching and burning and she noticed that her eyes were sticky when she woke up this morning.

Single best answer*
You are called to see a 78-year-old gentleman who lives alone. He has been unwell for a fortnight but didn't want to bother anybody; his last visit to the surgery was 15 years ago. He appears quite dehydrated and confused so you do some tests; the results are as follows:
    Glucose 50 mmol/l, sodium 135, potassium 5.0, urea 19, creatinine 145, plasma osmolalitiy 349 (278–305), Hb 18, WCC 17, Platelets 268, CRP 70.
    Urine dip: ketones ++, leucocytes +
What is the likely diagnosis?
    A dehydration secondary to urinary tract infection
    B dehydration secondary to self neglect
    C renal failure
    D diabetic ketoacidosis
    E hyperosmolar non-ketotic state
    F syndrome of inappropriate ADH secretion
    G nephrogenic diabetes incipidus

*© H Dawson, A Trigell. *EMQs for the MRCGP Paper 2: With Answers Discussed*. Radcliffe Medical Press, Oxford, 2005. Reproduced with the permission of the copyright holder.

Both assessments should be submitted or undertaken only in the final 6 months of training.

Video assessment

You may choose to produce a video solely for summative assessment, or submit your MRCGP tape. Full details of both are covered in *Chapter 19: The video*.

You may submit your video between the end of months six and nine as a GPR.

Simulated surgery project

Held in real surgeries in the LNR deanery area twice a year, this involves eight consultations of up to 10 minutes with trained 'simulators' playing patients. You have 5 minutes between consultations to complete a post-encounter sheet commenting on the consultation. The surgery lasts two and a half hours.

You must pass six consultations or you will need to undertake a further eight-patient surgery. If you fail this you will be referred to an expert panel.

You should bring your usual diagnostic equipment to the examination and a copy of the *BNF* or *MIMS*.

Applications should be made to the LNR deanery and forms are downloadable from the NOSA website. Your deanery will need to sign the application form to confirm funding (if you are not from the LNR deanery area).

Written work

This can either be the COGPED audit or a piece of work that fulfils the National Project Marking Schedule (NPMS) criteria. The work must relate to general practice and can be undertaken at any time throughout the 3 years of vocational training.

Choosing a topic can be an initial stumbling block. Unless you have a burning interest in something, ask your practice colleagues for ideas as they may need an audit doing for clinical governance purposes. Failing that, brainstorm with your VTS colleagues and read the GP press for hot topics. Whatever you choose, *keep it simple*. Ideally it should only take 10–12 hours work in total (*Box 17.4*). Your practice should provide all you need to carry out the audit.

Your written work must be submitted by the end of month nine of the registrar year. Specific and detailed instructions about the presentation and submission of your written piece of work are available from the NOSA website.

COGPED audit

See Chapter 21: Guidance for good professional practice – Clinical governance.

Audit is a core component of clinical governance* and the ability to complete an audit is considered a skill of minimum competence for GPs. You need to be

Box 17.4   Tips for your written submission

- Ensure you have protected time
- Give yourself adequate planning time before you start your data collection
- Enlist your trainer's help with planning, time-tabling, guidance on searching the literature, sample size, etc.
- Use a computer (database and simple graphics packages are essential)
- Do a literature search to help refine your criteria
- Ensure references are fully documented
- Use data easily available (e.g. on the practice computer database) to facilitate searches
- Never fabricate data

able to complete the 'audit cycle' and so need to start planning your audit very early on in the registrar year to give you an opportunity to do two data collections. The audit should be written up using the headings in *Box 17.5* and it must be under 3000 words.

Box 17.5   The COGPED audit criteria *Write up*

The following titles must be used and highlighted
Reason for the choice of audit
    Potential for change
    Relevance to the practice
Criterion/criteria chosen
    Relevant to audit subject and justifiable, e.g. current literature
Standards set
    Targets towards a standard with a suitable timescale
Preparation and planning
    Evidence of teamwork and adequate discussion where appropriate
Data collection (1)
    Results compared against a standard
Change(s) to be evaluated
    Actual example described
Data collection (2)
    Comparison with Data collection (1) and standard
Conclusions
    Summary of main issues learned

Under the NPMS, other, more creative, self-directed work can be submitted (*Box 17.6*). There is a 30-point marking schedule and 18 points are required to pass. This marking schedule is closely linked to the headings that should be used (*Box 17.7*).

Box 17.6   National Project Marking Schedule options for written work

Options for submission
- Questionnaire study or notes review
- Literature review
- Clinical case study
- Research study
- Proposal for new service in the practice
- Discussion paper

Box 17.7   National Project Marking Schedule

The following headings should be used in the write up:
- **Aim**
- **Literature** normally six or more references should be used
- **Method** the reader should have enough information to repeat what was done
- **Results** these should be clearly related to the aims
- **Discussion** evaluate your project; how does your project compare with previous work? what are the implications for practice?
- **Conclusion** summarise the main points; any potential for future work?

The structured trainer's report

This report, which is divided into six sections, gives your trainer specific guidance on the minimum standards they should expect from you (*Box 17.8*). Aim to complete:

- clinical skills in the first part of the year
- the patient care element as you prepare your video
- personal skills in the last 6 months when you should be more settled as an independent GP

Box 17.8 The structured trainer's report

Part 1 – Specific clinical skills
- Mental state examination
- Use of: auriscope, ophthalmoscope, sphygmomanometer, stethoscope, peak flow meter
- Vaginal examination
- Use of speculum
- Cervical smear
- Rectal examination
- Venous access
- i.m. and s.c. injections

Part 2 – Patient care
Making a diagnosis
- Communication skills
- Recognition of common physical, psychological and social problems
- Eliciting patients' beliefs, ideas, concerns and expectations
- Dealing with patients' life events and crises
- Proficient examination of each system and organ
- Undertakes examination with consideration of patients needs/feelings

Patient management
- Appropriate management of problems
- Management of emergency situations
- Care and support for patients and families
- Broad knowledge of all aspects of drugs

Clinical judgement
- Appropriate examination (including investigation)
- Appropriate response to requests for urgent attendance

Part 3 – Personal skills
Organisational skills
- Awareness of personal limitations, appropriate referral and delegation
- Time management
- Understanding of contractual obligations of a GP

Professional values
- Possession and application of ethical principles
- Maintenance of personal physical and mental health
- Accepting appropriate responsibility for patients, partners, colleagues *et al.*
- Establishes and maintains good relationships with patients
- Able to work with colleagues
- Keeps good records
- Demonstrates honesty

Personal and professional growth
- Identification of personal strengths and weaknesses

Reproduced with permission from the National Office for Summative Assessment.

Go through the trainer's report carefully with your trainer during your induction period. Your trainer should then fill in the report on a regular basis throughout the year, although they may need a little prompting from time to time. Your trainer must assess you by:

- observation, e.g. in joint surgeries, video, simulated patient situations
- case discussions
- tutorials

Your trainer can use evidence of competence from log books kept during your hospital training for some of the clinical skills.

Other 'recognised sources' who can assess some skills areas include:

- another GP
- consultant
- CPN
- pharmacist
- appropriately trained nurse
- family planning trainer
- receptionist

Submission of the trainer's report is at the end of month 11. It should be submitted to your local deanery with the signed VTR1 form (or equivalent).

By month 11 all registrars should have had plenty of opportunities to demonstrate the required skills. If your trainer has grave doubts about your ability to reach the required standard in all elements they will need to discuss it with you and inform your course organiser and deanery.

SOURCES AND FURTHER READING

1. National Office for Summative Assessment, www.nosa.org.uk
2. Royal College of General Practitioners, www.rcgp.org.uk
3. Joint Committee on Postgraduate Training for General Practice, www.jcptgp.org.uk
4. Postgraduate Medical Education and Training Board, www.pmetb.org.uk

Chapter 18
The MRCGP exam

INTRODUCTION

The MRCGP exam is an interesting assessment that encourages you to develop your own ideas about all aspects of general practice, health care and health politics. The exam should help you develop your critical faculties, structure your clinical thinking and begin to make sense of research papers in the major journals.

*See *Chapter 3: Working in the wider health service* – RCGP.

Passing the MRCGP exam is the main way to become a Member of the Royal College of General Practitioners* and should improve your job prospects. New GP trainers must hold the MRCGP but established trainers are not obliged to acquire it.

The exam is open to independent practitioners of general practice or those undergoing vocational training. Even if you pass the entire exam during your GPR year you won't be granted full college membership until you've received your certificate of completion of training from the JCPTGP (or PMETB).

This chapter is a summary of how to approach the exam. Check the college website for the latest regulations.

WHAT'S INVOLVED?

The exam is a four-part modular exam (*Box 18.1*) although you don't have to undertake all the modules in one sitting. The detailed syllabus has been guided by the GMC document '*Good Medical Practice*' and aims to test knowledge and skills that are thought to be important for a good general practitioner in the NHS today.

Each module is held twice a year. Three attempts at each module are permitted but all four modules must be passed within 3 years of application to pass overall, otherwise you have to start again. You need to make an application for the exam overall as well as for each individual module and you pay for each module (£295 each in 2005).

When applying to take the exam, you will need to provide a copy of your current GMC certificate, a photograph endorsed by a member or a fellow of the RCGP and established practitioners will need to provide evidence of their eligibility to practise. Before completing the exam you must submit evidence of your competence in cardiopulmonary resuscitation (*Box 18.2*).

Box 18.1   MRCGP examination modules

The written paper
- Modified essays and structured answers on management of common problems in general practice
- Critical reading: analysis and evaluation of published papers and extracts
- Knowledge of general practice literature
- 12 or so equally marked short answer questions
- 3 hours with normally 30 minutes added for reading

The multiple choice paper
- Up to 250 multiple choice questions in a variety of formats
- 3 hour paper, machine-marked, no negative marking
- Covers:
  - medicine 65%
  - administration and management 15%
  - research, epidemiology and statistics 20%

Assessment of consulting skills: video or simulated surgery
- Video recording of self-selected consultations
Or
- Simulated surgery consulting with a sequence of actors playing patients with defined roles:
  - Held twice a year
  - Only available to those with insuperable difficulties in making a video

The oral exam (viva)
- Two consecutive 20 minute orals
- Each conducted by two examiners
- Emphasis on decision making and the professional values that underpin this
- Approximately five topics covered in each
- Covers:
  - Care of patients
  - Working with colleagues
  - Social role of general practice
  - Doctor's personal responsibilities

Box 18.2   Cardio-pulmonary resuscitation performance test

Certificates provided in MRCGP exam regulations book/RCGP website
Valid 3 years from date of signing
Submitted before you complete the exam

Candidates must be competent in:
- basic life support, including use of oropharyngeal airway and pocket mask
- use of external automated defibrillator in a patient with a shockable rhythm

Assessment by A&E or anaesthetic consultant, GP with special interest in CPR, Resuscitation Training Officer, St John's Ambulance, etc.

Holders of ALS certificate issued within last 3 years exempt

WHEN TO SIT IT

Processing the current literature and mastering critical appraisal requires a lot of work so you may choose to defer at least some modules until after you have finished your registrar year.

Some choose to do the exam immediately after being a GPR and locum work can provide some flexibility for studying. Other GPs prefer to leave it until later, but you run the risk of never finding the ideal time.

There are two sittings a year, usually May–July and October–December. Applications have to be in several months before the exam; early February for the summer sitting and late August for the winter sitting.

HOW TO APPROACH IT

The following will help your preparations:

- Read both GP and non-GP texts. Anything with a remotely health and social care, ethical, organisational, educational or political flavour will be useful and will keep your mind ticking over. Include the daily press and novels.
- Learn and practice the skill of critical appraisal; how to read and analyse a paper. Some books and courses may be helpful and your VTS may run sessions devoted to this.

- Go through the current literature and identify the 'hot topics'. Use the GP press as well as the standard journals. Books and courses are available.
- Keep summaries of key facts, main reference papers and contentious issues.
- Practice viva questions.
- Use the past written papers with examiners comments available on the RCGP website to practice for the written paper.
- Develop an approach to the written questions which can be used to answer questions on clinical problems, practice management, professional values and broader political themes. It may be helpful to discuss this amongst your colleagues in a study group.
- You may be able to organise teaching and assessment for CPR with a group from the VTS or through your practice which needs to organise training for members of the practice as a requirement of the GMS contract.
- Speak to GPs who have done the exam. Ask them about the questions they were asked as many themes are revisited in subsequent exam sittings.

MRCGP study group

A study group can be an excellent way of focusing on the exam. You can share ideas and sources of information and it can provide you with a way of practising examination technique and reviewing videos. Aim for a group of between three and six members. The VTS is likely to be the best source of registrars interested in a group. If you are attempting the exam after your training then contact the local VTS; a study group may well welcome a more experienced GP.

Aim to meet at least 3 months in advance of the exam, perhaps fortnightly to start with then weekly closer to the exam. Spend time planning how you will run the meetings and prepare a list of topics. Include clinical problems and broader general practice themes.

Each member could focus on an individual topic, research the information and then produce a handout summary for everyone.

Aim to cover:

- a revision of basic facts
- new developments
- application to clinical practice
- summaries of key papers
- future developments
- contentious points

Current literature and 'hot topics'

The clinical 'hot topics' are likely to come from papers published in the main journals (*Box 18.3*) in the last 18 months. Other important studies are likely to be summarised in these journals. Recently published research papers are often summarised and commented on in the GP press so it can be worth reading before (and if) you confront the original research paper. You will need

Box 18.3   Sources for 'hot topics'

Books See *Sources and further reading*

Journals
- *British Medical Journal* (pay particular attention to 'theme' issues)
- *British Journal of General Practice*
- *Drug and Therapeutics Bulletin*

Medical Press
e.g. *Pulse, Doctor, GP*
may summarise key findings of research and discuss developments in general practice

Courses
Look in the *BMJ* and *BJGP*, and ask your colleagues about recommended 'hot topics' courses

Others
- National guidelines, e.g. NICE, Scottish Intercollegiate Guideline Network (SIGN), National Service Frameworks (NSFs)
- RCGP occasional papers
- Seminal papers on important topics
- *Clinical Evidence* – a continually update source of the latest evidence. Produced by BMJ Publishing. Also available online, www.clinicalevidence.com

to be aware of seminal past research papers that have influenced key developments in practice.

Questions on 'hot topics' do not only focus on clinical developments but may cover anything new affecting general practice such as service developments, government directives, new ethical guidance, changes to contracts and working conditions in general practice. Again much of this is written about in the medical press and journals.

You should be able to mention references from reputable journals in your answers but it is not essential to quote results and references precisely. In the written paper it is more important that you make the examiner aware that you understand the meaning and relevance of a piece of research rather than be able to quote the exact source.

MRCGP courses

*See Chapter 5: Contract and finances – Study leave and study leave reimbursements.

Courses may focus on all or one of the modules. Fees may be reimbursable from your educational allowance if you are a registrar or from your Higher Professional Education (HPE) allowance if you are newly qualified*.

The RCGP and its regional faculties run courses as do many other independent organisations. Look at the RCGP website, your deanery website and look in the *BMJ* and *BJGP* for advertised courses.

The video

Preparation for this is covered in the next chapter.

MEMBERSHIP BY ASSESSMENT OF PERFORMANCE

Membership by Assessment of Performance (MAP) provides an alternative means of achieving college membership. It is intended primarily for established GPs who don't have the time available for the intensive study involved in the examination. Those eligible must have at least 5 years independent practice and have been working at least three sessions a week in general practice in the year before application. MAP shares with the exam the requirement of assessment of consultation skills by video or simulated surgery. However, the other skills are tested by completion of a workbook and a day-long practice visit by external assessors. It costs the same as undertaking the exam but may take several months or years to complete. Bear it in mind if you vowed never to do another medical exam after summative assessment!

SOURCES AND FURTHER READING

1. Royal College of General Practitioners, www.rcgp.org.uk
2. Resuscitation Council guidance on basic life support and automated external defibrillators, www.resus.org.uk/pages/guide.htm
3. Acheson P., Daniels R., Neumegen G. *Practice Papers for the MRCGP Written Exam.* PasTest Ltd, 2002.
4. Dawson H., Trigell, A. *EMQs for the MRCGP Paper 2: with Answers Discussed.* Radcliffe Medical Press, 2005.
5. Field S., Gear S. *The Complete MRCGP Study Guide.* Radcliffe Medical Press, Oxford, 2003.
6. Kilburn J. *Answer Plans for the MRCGP 2nd edition.* Scion Publishing Ltd, 2004.
7. Greenhalgh T. *How to Read a Paper.* BMJ Publishing, 2004.
8. Stacey E. and Toun Y. *Critical Reading Questions for the MRCGP 2nd edition.* Scion Publishing Ltd, 2005.
9. Website produced by Ese Stacey including details of courses, reading materials, www.mrcgpexam.co.uk
10. Kilburn J. *Hot Topics in General Practice 6th edition.* Scion Publishing Ltd, 2005.
11. Naidoo P., Davy A. *Concepts and Answers for the MRCGP Oral Exam.* Scion Publishing Ltd, 2005.

Chapter 19
The Video

INTRODUCTION

Videos of the consultation have become an inescapable part of formal GP training. Although reviewing video recordings of your consultations is a very useful educational process, producing an edited tape of consultations suitable for exam purposes with a pertinent commentary can be time consuming and anxiety provoking. This chapter concentrates only on producing videos for examination purposes. You can find out more about consultation techniques from other sources*.

*See *Chapter 7: The consultation: survival tips for the new GP* – Sources and further reading.

†See *Chapter 17: Summative assessment* and *Chapter 18: The MRCGP exam.*

Both summative assessment and the MRCGP exam include evaluation of consulting skills and reviewing videoed consultations plays an important part of these assessments, although there are alternative ways of being assessed†. Check the latest guidelines and exam regulations produced by the National Office for Summative Assessment (NOSA) and the Royal College of General Practitioners (RCGP).

Although seeing and hearing yourself on screen may be excruciating, the more you do, the easier it gets. Start to video consultations well before your submission deadline (from month 2 in the registrar year). This will help you get used to the process and technicalities even if you are not yet confident about your consulting skills. When you feel ready, start video-taping with the requirements of both summative assessment and the MRCGP exam in mind.

PRACTICALITIES

Basic equipment

Training Practices are obliged to provide all the necessary equipment for a registrar's summative assessment requirements including video equipment (*Box 19.1*).

Setting up the camera

Familiarise yourself with the basic workings of the camera. Get a demonstration and read the instruction booklet. Make a short test recording with a member of practice staff *each* time you set up your equipment (*Box 19.2*).

Preparing the consulting room

Reduce clutter on your desk and ensure any shelves aren't bare. Arrange the furniture so both you and the patient are visible. Ensure the examination couch is out of view or keep the camera running with the lens cap on when examining patients.

Box 19.1   Video equipment

- Video camera, ideally with:
    - Tripod or wall mounting facility
    - Lens cap/shutter with on-going sound recording
    - Remote control
    - Built-in and remote microphone
    - Date, timer counter with on-screen display (essential for summative assessment)
    - Playback on the camera
- Several blank tapes for the camera
- VHS tapes which may be supplied by the deanery for summative assessment
- VCR player – to edit/record from the camera.
- Consent forms (photocopy at least 50 to start with)
- Practice information leaflet should be available and should make reference to videoing/training
- Clipboard and pens at reception

Box 19.2   Setting up the camera

- Ensure both you and the patient are in the frame
- Don't have the camera facing direct light/windows (close blinds and use artificial lighting)
- Check sound quality – use an external microphone if necessary
- Close windows and turn off fans
- Ensure date/timer display are on
- Ensure you have enough film in the camera

PLANNING

Organising video surgeries

Start by video-taping a few consultations in a surgery then plan to do a weekly video surgery once you are more confident. Vary your video day as Friday afternoon general practice can be very different from Wednesday mornings.

You will need to block out appointments or increase your appointment time for video surgeries. Good consulting and technical hitches take time and some patients may use consultation time discussing the video process itself.

Bear in mind that submitted consultations should ideally be no longer than 15 minutes (see *Box 19.6*).

Reception staff are crucial to the smooth running of the video surgery and you should involve them fully. Be sure they understand why you are videoing; this should help them to encourage, but not bully, patients to consent (see below). Receptionists should hand out the consent form with a pen before the consultation but it is usually easier for you to get the post-consultation consent. Ask for interruptions to be minimised.

Aim to tape at least four times as many consultations as you'll need to submit to give you a good pool to select from. Many of your recordings may be unsuitable for technical, not clinical, reasons (see *Box 19.3*).

Consent and maintaining confidentiality

Consultations may only be filmed with explicit informed consent. Most patients are happy to be filmed to help with teaching and training but the opportunity to decline should always be offered. Ideally, patients should be informed of your intention to video the surgery when they book the appointment.

Consent forms must be signed **both before and after the consultation.** The NOSA and RCGP have forms which are downloadable from their websites (and can be used interchangeably). The signed form should be kept in the patient's medical record. You should write that a consultation was video recorded in the patient's notes. Anyone accompanying a patient who appears in the video should also give consent.

Confidentiality, the reason for the video, and who will be viewing the tape should be emphasised. Some patients, such as non-English speakers, refugees and those with mental illness, may need extra explanation (or you may think it is better not to record in these circumstances).

The recordings and tapes should be stored with the same security as medical records. You should leave them in a locked cupboard or drawer. All recordings should be destroyed as soon as possible and definitely within 3 years.

Taping the consultation

You must tape the entire consultation. Be ready to turn off the camera at any point at the patient's request. You can film 'non-intimate' examinations but bear in mind you are not being assessed on your clinical examination skills and a poor technique might negatively influence examiners so it may be best to perform all examinations 'off camera'. Intimate examinations should certainly not be seen but remember to take off the lens cap or open the curtains afterwards. You must keep the camera running during an examination. You may decide to tape the entire surgery leaving the tape running, but this can waste tape and is tedious to review.

Pitfalls

However well your surgeries seem to go there are often unpleasant surprises when you come to review your tapes. Learn from our mistakes (*Box 19.3*).

Box 19.3   Video pitfalls

- Overbooking video clinics
- Forgetting to put on the timer
- Running out of tape mid-consultation
- Catching only part of the patient's or doctor's face
- Seeing too much of an intimate examination
- Lighting and noise 'pollution'
- Failure to get post-consultation consent
- Overlong good quality consultations
- Recording over tapes you haven't yet reviewed
- Starting to video shortly before the submission deadline, so only having a small pool of consultations to choose from

---

Reviewing your taped consultations

You need to have a method of indexing and storing your tapes as there is nothing worse than recording over a consultation that you felt was suitable for submission. Review your tapes regularly and soon after you make them as hours of accumulated surgeries to review is a daunting task. View your consultations on your own to start with and then ask your trainer, mentor or other colleagues for advice on selection for submission for summative assessment and the MRCGP exam. Showing videos to the VTS or your study group can also provide some invaluable feedback.

REQUIREMENTS FOR SUMMATIVE ASSESSMENT AND MRCGP VIDEOS

Registrars can submit the same video for both summative assessment and MRCGP via the 'Single Route Assessment'. You need to decide early on in the registrar year if you are going to apply for this as you must indicate which assessment of your consulting skills you intend to undergo on your summative assessment application form.

A pass in the consulting skills module of the MRCGP is a sufficient demonstration of competence for summative assessment. If you do the single route and you do not pass the MRCGP consulting module, your video will be automatically entered into the summative assessment process.

As the MRCGP video criteria are more demanding, some registrars prefer to complete the summative assessment video and submit this before tackling the requirements of MRCGP at a later date. However, the NOSA recommends the single route as the preferred method of assessment.

If you are using the same tape for both, send your tape and paperwork to your deanery by the specified dates and they will forward it to the RCGP examiners. If you fail the MRCGP video module, it will be returned to the deanery who will then assess it for the summative assessment criteria.

The Wessex Faculty of the RCGP has produced a DVD showing consultations that satisfy the RCGP performance criteria which may be a practical guide as to what the RCGP is after.

PREPARING YOUR FINAL TAPE FOR SUBMISSION

Don't underestimate how long this can take. You need to:

- review hours of taped surgeries
- select technically and clinically suitable consultations
- ensure consultations demonstrate the skills being tested (*Box 19.4* and *19.5*) so don't use 'no challenge' consultations. Try to use 'first presentations' as follow-up consultations do not always provide you with the scope to pass all the criteria for the MRCGP exam
- get at least one independent assessment of your selections
- edit on to a single VHS tape with the MRCGP exam consultations first if appropriate
- make at least one copy for yourself
- analyse the content of each consultation and complete the summary forms
- complete the log of the tape with accurate timing

Box 19.4   Summative assessment: competencies to be demonstrated

- Identify the reasons for the patient's attendance
- Take appropriate steps to investigate the problems presented
- Organise a suitable management plan
- Reach an agreement with the patient on diagnosis and treatment
- Demonstrate an understanding of what was going on in the consultation (in the logbook)

The consultations should be free of any major errors or a series of minor errors that may cause the patient inconvenience or embarrassment

---

Box 19.5   MRCGP video: competencies to be demonstrated

There are 14 performance criteria; 10 are pass criteria, 4 are merit criteria (marked *)

In order to pass you need to have demonstrated each pass criteria 4 times

Discover the reasons for the patient's attendance:
1: the doctor is seen to encourage the patient's contribution at appropriate points in the consultation
2: the doctor is seen to respond to signals (cues) that lead to a deeper understanding of the problem*
3: the doctor uses appropriate psychological and social information to place the complaint(s) in context
4: the doctor explores the patient's health understanding

Define the clinical problem(s):
5: the doctor obtains sufficient information to include or exclude likely relevant significant conditions
6: the physical/mental examination chosen is likely to confirm or disprove hypotheses that could reasonably have been formed *or* is designed to address a patient's concern
7: the doctor appears to make a clinically appropriate working diagnosis

Explain the problem(s) to the patient:
8: the doctor explains the problem or diagnosis in appropriate language
9: the doctor's explanation incorporates some or all of the patient's health beliefs*
10: the doctor specifically seeks to confirm the patient's understanding of the diagnosis*

Address the patient's problem(s):
11: the management plan (including any prescription) is appropriate for the working diagnosis, reflecting a good understanding of modern accepted medical practice
12: the patient is given the opportunity to be involved in significant management decisions

Make effective use of the consultation:
13: in prescribing the doctor takes steps to enhance concordance, by exploring and responding to the patient's understanding of the treatment*
14: the doctor specifies the conditions and interval for follow-up or review

Box 19.6   Comparison of video requirements

Summative assessment	MRCGP exam
See website www.nosa.org.uk for up to date guidelines	See website www.rcgp.org.uk for up to date guidelines
Apply via local deanery (and RCGP if single route)	Apply to RCGP
Two hours of complete consultations, minimum eight consultations. If single route, the first seven must be suitable for the MRCGP exam	Seven complete consultations
Maximum 20 minutes per consultation. MRCGP examiners will only assess first 15 mins if making single route application	Maximum 20 minutes per consultation. Only first 15 minutes of consultation will be assessed
In English (Welsh if patient's preference but other consultations must be in English). Logbook must be in English	In English
Good sound and picture quality (with doctor and patient clearly visible)	As summative assessment
No intimate examinations to be seen (sound recording to continue)	As summative assessment
No clinical content specified	Must include • one consultation with child under 10 years • one with significant psychological or social dimension
Use standard summative assessment/MRCGP consent form and file in patients notes	As summative assessment

Box 19.6 *continued*

Summative assessment	MRCGP exam
Standard VHS format. Date and time must be clearly visible on each consultation (and correspond to logbook)	Standard VHS format
Submit with logbook, logbook summary (two copies if single route) and video declaration form signed by yourself and trainer. Hand deliver / send by recorded delivery to the deanery	Submit with logbook and summary to RCGP
Submit by end of month nine (but not before month 6)	Check RCGP website for deadlines
Pass or fail, but re-submission possible	Pass with merit, pass or fail

For the final tape you may wish to record a short introduction such as: 'My name is Dr .... and I am making this recording for summative assessment and the MRCGP exam'.

Go through the final checklists for summative assessment or the MRCGP exam before submitting the tape. Ensure you have numbered the consent forms appropriately, included one for each consultation and filled in the summaries legibly. Deliver the final product (in a protective padded envelope) personally, or by registered post or courier and then breathe a huge sigh of relief until the results come through!

SOURCES AND FURTHER READING

1. Royal College of General Practitioners, www.rcgp.org.uk
2. National Office for Summative Assessment, www.nosa.org.uk
3. GMC. *Making and Using Visual and Audio Recordings of Patients*, 2003. www.gmc-uk.org
4. *Consultation Skills for the MRCGP DVD*. Available from Carol White, Wessex Faculty RCGP, Andover Memorial Hospital, Charlton Road, Andover SP10 3LB Tel: 01264 355005; Email: cwhite@rcgp.org.uk.

Chapter 20
Appraisal and revalidation

INTRODUCTION

Appraisal and revalidation have been introduced in part due to poor morale amongst some doctors and a need for the profession to demonstrate safe self-regulation after the medical disasters of the Bristol heart cases, retention of body parts in Alder Hey and Harold Shipman.

On a more positive note, appraisal should feed into a formalised system that supports and encourages doctors' ongoing development and learning and forms part of a clinical governance-led NHS.

This chapter aims to summarise what you need to know to get through appraisal and how to get the most out of the experience without being over-whelmed by the process.

The guidance for revalidation was not available at the time of going to press and so this chapter explains the themes of the process only and points you in the right direction for up to date guidance.

APPRAISAL

There are a number of definitions of appraisal as applied to the NHS (see *Box 20.1*).

Box 20.1   Definitions of appraisal

Conlon, *BMJ*, 2003
'a structured process of self reflection'

DOH, 2003
'Ongoing, two-way process involving reflection on an individual's performance, identification of education needs and planning for personal development.'

Appraisal for GPs from the School of Health and Related Research
'– exploring role, expectations, negotiating relative priorities, and setting and aligning individual and organisational objectives at local level
– reviewing progress towards achieving previously agreed objectives and agreeing future objectives
– recognising, acknowledging and valuing achievements
– exploring what is needed from the organisation to help and support the individual in making the best contribution they can'

The aims of GP appraisal are:

- regular review of a doctor's work
- production of an individual Personal Development Plan (see *Box 20.2*)
- optimal use of skills and resources to achieve delivery of medical care locally
- identify resource needs locally
- meet some of the requirements for revalidation

Box 20.2 Personal development plan

A tool to help describe personal development objectives and the development activities designed to help achieve them.

It should take account of:
- professional development needs
- practice requirements
- personal ambitions

Stages in preparing the plan:
- where are you now – current level of competence
- specific things you want to achieve
- what level of achievement you are aiming for
- how you are going to go about achieving your goals
- when and how you are going to review your progress

Appraisal is based on the GMC components of good medical care (see *Box 20.3*). It is not designed or intended to identify poor performance; if performance problems do come out during appraisal they must be dealt with outside the appraisal.

Box 20.3 GMC components of good medical practice

Good clinical care
Maintaining good medical practice
Relationships with patients
Working with colleagues
Teaching and training
Probity
Health

Your GP appraiser has the same duty as any doctor under the GMC '*Duties of a Doctor*' to 'act quickly to protect patients from risk if you have good reason to believe that you or a colleague may not be fit to practice'. It should be very rare that a previous unknown issue of poor performance arises in an appraisal.

Appraisers

For an appraisal system to work the appraisee must have trust and respect for their appraiser and the appraiser must be properly trained.

In primary care, GPs appraise each other. The PCO has a responsibility to ensure enough local GPs are trained as appraisers to provide appraisal in their area without a small number of GPs being overburdened with the work.

The appraisal training usually takes one to two days. Appraisers should then meet regularly for ongoing training and support.

The PCO pays their appraisers for each appraisal they do. If after your appraisal you are not happy about your appraiser, feed this back to the PCO. Ask to have another appraiser the following year.

The appraisal process

The appraisal process involves gathering information from day to day activities and self reflection and a discussion based on these at the annual appraisal interview. This leads to the identification of learning and development needs for your PDP for the following year.

The information for discussion for the appraisal interview should be kept in your appraisal folder; this can be on paper, disc or online.

There are five forms to be completed (*Box 20.4*).

Forms 1 and 2 provide factual information about you and your job and take a few minutes to complete.

Form 3 is the main content of your appraisal and is based on the GMC guidelines '*Good Medical Practice*' (*Box 20.3*) and may take several hours to complete.

Each section will ask you about your skills and limitations and ask you to reflect on your work. If this is not your first appraisal you will be asked to reflect back on your appraisal the previous year.

Box 20.4   Forms for appraisal

Form 1   Basic details
Form 2   Current medical activities
Form 3   Material for appraisal
Form 4   Summary of the appraisal discussion and PDP
Form 5   Detailed confidential account of the appraisal interview

---

You should aim to back up your information with documents. Suitable things to keep over the year to include are audits, significant event analysis, meetings, teaching events, teaching commitments. You can either keep paper or computer documents as the year goes on (see *Box 20.5*).

Form 4 is completed during the appraisal interview. The appraisee and appraiser must agree on action points which constitute the basis of the PDP (*Box 20.2*).

Ideally you should agree on four or five objectives. Be realistic in what you can achieve and use SMART (*Box 20.6*) for all your objectives (*Box 20.7*).

For qualified GPs **Form 4** is forwarded to the PCT. GPRs keep all the paperwork from their appraisal themselves.

Form 5 is an optional form for GPs to fill out confidentially after their appraisal for a personal record of that year's appraisal meeting

---

Box 20.5   Examples of things to collect for your appraisal

Audits
Significant event analysis
Examples of reflective learning
Examples of online learning activities
Timetable of practice and local meetings attended
Courses attended with your assessment
Puns and Dens (Patient's Unmet Needs, Doctor's Educational Needs)
Summary of a complaint you were involved in and your learning outcomes
Personal prescribing data
Personal referral data
Electronic CME modules completed
Details of research

Box 20.6   SMART for your appraisal objectives

Specific
Measurable
Attainable
Realistic
Timed

The process of form filling and the appraisal interview is supposed to take between 4 and 6.5 hours. You should be given at least 2 months notice of your appraisal date and some protected time for this work.

Try not to let the appraisal process become overwhelming, keep supporting documents you collect over the year accessible and don't aim for perfect form filling. Remember the whole process is supposed to be for your benefit. The vast majority of GPs who have undergone appraisal have found it a rewarding process.

Appraisal for registrars

All doctors in training are required to participate in the appraisal process but the emphasis of their appraisal should be on their education as opposed to the self reflection and personal development of trained GPs. Appraisal is in addition to summative assessment requirements and should take place towards the end of the registrar year. It is the responsibility of the registrar to complete the forms and gather the information, but your trainer should help you organise the appraisal.

Outcomes from the registrar appraisal should be:

- familiarity with the NHS appraisal process
- an educational appraisal
- a PDP to take into the next year

Registrars should keep all documents relating to the appraisal as evidence for revalidation.

Registrars are usually appraised by a GP trainer other than their own who has also received appraisal training.

IT support for appraisal

The appraisal forms can be completed online on the NHS appraisal website www.appraisals.nhs.uk. Once you have signed it off it will link directly to your PCO appraisal administrator and your appraiser will be able to access the information before your interview.

There are websites which provide online learning materials and record your learning activity. This can be used as supporting information*.

*See Appendix 1: Useful websites.

REVALIDATION

In future all doctors who wish to practise medicine in the UK will need to hold a licence to practise. The privileges currently associated with GMC registration, for example, employment in the NHS and the right to prescribe, will attach to this licence. To retain this licence, doctors will have to 'revalidate' by demonstrating, on a regular basis, that they remain up to date and fit to practise.

The purpose of revalidation is to ensure that patients can have confidence that their doctors are competent and abide by high ethical standards. It has three broad aims:

- to encourage all doctors to reflect on their work, using evidence gathered through audit and in other ways
- to update what being registered and being qualified means, by shifting the emphasis away from being qualified, to being up to date and fit to practise
- to replace the 'management by exception' approach that has been in place since 1858, by introducing regular confirmation that there are no significant concerns about a doctor's practice and that the doctor is up to date and fit to practise

At the time of going to press the implementation of the licence and the precise definition of the model for revalidation were on hold pending the outcome of Sir Liam Donaldson's review of the recommendations in the Shipman Inquiry's 5th report.

You should, however, continue to participate in appraisal, collect information showing you are practising in line with the GMC's guidance on 'Good Medical Practice' and watch the GMC's website www.gmc-uk.org for the latest details on the implementation and timing of the license to practice and revalidation.

Make sure the GMC always has your up to date address.

SOURCES AND FURTHER READING

1. Board of Science and Education. *Appraisal: a Guide for Medical Practitioners.* BMA, November 2003.
2. NHS Appraisal, www.appraisals.nhs.uk
3. Department of Health, www.dh.gov.uk; www.revalidationuk.info
4. London Deanery. *Appraisal for Doctors in Training*, www.londondeanery.ac.uk
5. GMC, www.gmc-uk.org
6. GMC. *Licensing and Revalidation Formal Guidance for Doctors.* GMC **draft**, September 2004.
7. *Appraisal for General Practitioners Working in Scotland* available on, www.rcgp-scotland.org.uk
8. RCGP, *Scotland Revalidation Folder*, www.nes.scot.nhs.uk
9. Zwanenberg T. Revalidation: the purpose needs to be clear. *BMJ*, **328**: 684–686, 2004.

Chapter 21
Guidance for good professional practice

INTRODUCTION

Even if you are extremely clinically astute and conscientious, problems can arise from poor communication or system failures. Worse still, you can be tripped up simply because you are not aware of some of the legal stipulations.

This chapter and *Chapter 22* should help you avoid mistakes in patient care and make you aware of some of your legal responsibilities.

Legal stipulations are derived from statutes, e.g. Data Protection Act 1988, or from case law where the principles used to judge one specific case can be applied generally to an area of clinical practice. There are also codes of conduct or statements of professional responsibility issued by the GMC.

There are frequent changes in the law and guidance produced. Keep yourself up to date by:

- reading GMC guidance booklets
- reading information provided by your medical protection organisation and reviewing their website
- keeping an eye out in the medical press
- buying a text on the legal aspects of medical practice

If problems do arise, discuss them early with your colleagues within the practice. Have a low threshold for contacting your medical protection organisation for advice on any legal, ethical or professional practice matter.

The principles and legal requirements discussed in this chapter apply to the law in England and Wales only so check variations in Scotland and Northern Ireland.

YOUR RESPONSIBILITIES

Duties of a doctor

There are 14 key principles which summarise the responsibilities of a doctor. You must comply with these as an obligation of registration with the GMC (See *Box 21.1*).

Familiarise yourself with '*Good Medical Practice for GPs*'; a key document produced by the RCGP and the General Practitioners Committee.

Reducing risks in clinical management

A few key principles:

- Keep full, legible and up-to-date notes. Carefully document any clinical encounter, including telephone calls. Remember to date and sign entries. Take particular care in documenting difficult, emergency and OOH encounters.
- Keep patients and any health professionals involved in their care fully informed, unless the patient requests otherwise.

- Be meticulous when you prescribe*.   *See *Chapter 8: Prescribing.*
- Adopt accepted practice; follow guidelines when applicable, especially evidence-based ones.
- Act within your limitations; look things up, ask for help or refer as necessary.
- If you delegate then be sure that the person is up to the task.

You should practice defensible, not defensive medicine. Defensive medicine can be exhausting, inefficient and damaging to the doctor–patient relationship.

PRACTICE RESPONSIBILITIES

Rigorous systems should be in place for:

- repeat prescriptions
- reviewing results
- ensuring patient follow up
- dealing with incoming patient information
- passing on messages
- making routine and urgent referrals
- flagging up important clinical information, e.g allergies

These systems should have been devised with the staff working in the relevant areas and reviewed regularly. You should have an introduction to the practice systems in your induction period*; let the practice manager know if you feel a practice system could be improved.

*See *Chapter 4: Starting in the practice.*

CLINICAL GOVERNANCE

This was introduced in 1999 by the DOH in order to maintain high standards and safeguard quality within the NHS. All health professionals should be involved in clinical governance and PCOs and practices should have an appointed clinical governance lead (*Box 21.2*).

In practice, clinical governance means practices must develop health and safety protocols, organise regular audits and review adverse events amongst other things. With the support of PCOs, local guideline initiatives, audit and educational groups, practices in a given area can work towards common goals and standards.

UNDERSTANDING CONSENT

A patient's consent is required in any medical interaction (*Box 21.3*) although the nature of consent and the documentation required as evidence of the consent depends on the actual situation.

Box 21.2　Components of clinical governance

Clinical and organisational audit	Reviews whether a process conforms to a predetermined standard
Risk management	Aims to reduce the likelihood of adverse events affecting staff and patients
Significant event analysis	Ensures that lessons are learnt from mistakes or system failures
Evidence-based practice	Good quality evidence to support clinical practice
Quality improvement	Monitoring and measuring performance against standards
Personal and organisational development	Development and training
Assessment / appraisal of staff	All health care professionals should undergo regular assessment focusing on performance and development
Obtaining patients' and users' views	Develop partnership with the public. Includes procedures for complaints
Measures for tackling under-performance	Practices should have systems for managing under-performance either internally or with external support

Box 21.3   Clinical situations for which consent must be sought

- All clinical examinations
- Investigations including simple blood tests
- Treatments including injections, minor surgery procedures, radiographic procedures and major surgery
- Passing on medical information to any third party, e.g. relatives, spouse, employers or insurance company
- Others sitting in on the consultation, i.e. students, trainees, other health professionals, patients' friends, relatives, translators, health advocates
- Photographing, video- or audio-taping patients
- Entry into clinical trials
- Intimate examinations, i.e. rectal, genital and breast
  - always offer a chaperone
  - explain the procedure and why it is necessary
  - be prepared to stop the procedure at any time if the patient requests
  - provide privacy for undressing and redressing

Failure to obtain appropriate consent can lead to a claim for and potential recovery of damages. A few situations exist where consent is not required: treatment authorised under the Mental Health Act, some immigration and psychiatric examinations, and treatment ordered by a court.

For termination of pregnancy or sterilisation procedures consent is required from the patient only. It is good practice to seek to involve the patient's partner in the discussion but only with the patient's full agreement.

Nature and validity of consent

Three conditions must be satisfied to ensure consent is valid:

1. the patient must have the capacity to give consent (see *Competence* below)
2. the patient must have sufficient information to make an informed choice
3. the consent must be given voluntarily

Consent may be implied, such as by presentation at the surgery for a medical examination, or given expressly. You should be careful not to misinterpret a patient's apparent compliance as consent. The patient should always be fully informed before they can give consent so you must explain any procedures and treatments you intend to carry out. They should be aware of alternative options to the treatment offered, including no treatment. Confirm with them that they have enough information to make a decision and document your discussion.

Oral consent should be sufficient for most procedures carried out in general practice such as venesection, but for more complex procedures, typically minor surgery, you may wish to obtain written consent. Although there are actually few situations where it is legally imperative to obtain written consent, e.g. for some fertility treatments, documented consent provides some evidence that it has been obtained and may be useful should there be a future challenge.

Competence (or the capacity to make decisions)

Every adult should be assumed to be competent unless proven otherwise. For an adult to be considered competent they must be able to understand, believe and retain the information which is relevant to the decision, and be able to weigh it in the balance and make a decision.

Children, 'Fraser competence' and parental responsibility

Young people aged 16–17 years can consent to treatment as if they were adults. A child under 16 years can consent to medical treatment themselves if they are 'Fraser competent' (formerly Gillick competent), i.e. they have sufficient understanding and intelligence to enable them to understand fully what is proposed and any alternative options. A competent child of any age can also refuse treatment, but this can be overridden by a parent or a court if it is considered to be in the child's best interests (different rules apply in Scotland). You should seek legal advice if ever you find yourself in such a situation.

Several individuals can consent on behalf of a child:

- anyone with parental responsibility as set out by the 1989 Children Act (see *Box 21.4*)
- a court if necessary

Where contraceptive advice and treatment are concerned, young people under 16 years can be seen and treated without the consent of their parents if the treating doctor feels they are competent. You should always encourage parental involvement but it is not obligatory, and you should reassure the young person that they will be seen in confidence.

- The child's parents if married at the time of conception or birth
- The child's mother
- If unmarried at time of conception or birth, the child's father can gain responsibility
  - if he signs the child's birth certificate
  - if he subsequently marries the mother
  - via a court order
  - via a responsibility agreement
- Legally appointed guardian
- Local authority if child protection proceedings are ongoing
- A person in whose favour the court has made a residence order concerning the child

Refusal of consent

A competent adult is entitled to refuse treatment, investigations or hospital admission. A competent pregnant woman can refuse any treatment even if it would be harmful to the foetus.

If a competent patient's choice seems irrational to you, or not what you would consider to be in their best interests, then you should review whether they have enough information on which to base their decision. You have a duty to explain fully all the implications of rejecting the proposed inter-vention and offer the best available alternative to which they will agree. If they still refuse then respect their wishes.

*See *Chapter 10: Referrals* – Patients refusing emergency referral and *Chapter 11: Investigations and results* – Patients refusing investigations.

Document the interaction fully*.

Treating incompetent adults ('best interests' principle)

Currently no one can give consent on behalf of an incompetent or mentally incapacitated adult in England and Wales. However, the patient can be treated in their 'best interests' without their consent. Any such treatment should be limited to that which saves life, ensures improvement or prevents deterio-ration in their physical or mental health. This decision should take into account any advance statements†, knowledge of their background and input from those who know them well. In Scotland, the Adults with Incapacity Act 2000, allows a welfare attorney to be appointed. These individuals can make decisions about the health and welfare of patients who lack capacity.

†See *Chapter 22: Clinical issues with legal stipulations* – Advance directives.

The Mental Capacity Bill which is before Parliament at the time of writing should allow attorneys to be appointed in England and Wales. They will have what is known as a lasting power of attorney and will be able to make decisions about financial, health and personal welfare for an adult if they later become incapacitated*.

*See Chapter 22: Clinical issues with legal stipulations – Power of attorney.

Emergency situations where consent cannot be sought

In such situations the 'best interests' principle above should be followed, with treatment limited to the immediately necessary. You should tell the patient what has been done and why as soon as they are sufficiently recovered.

Where parents refuse consent for a child in an emergency situation but a doctor considers it in the child's best interest to go ahead, then the child can be treated. Again, seek legal advice in such situations.

Temporary incompetence

Patients may be treated in their 'best interests' without their consent in situations of temporary incompetence such as severe pain or panic induced by fear.

Examinations for medico-legal purposes

Such examinations for the police, or a solicitor still require a patient's consent unless there is a court order or authority under the Police and Criminal Evidence Act. Again, always seek advice from your protection organisation.

CONFIDENTIALITY

Confidentiality is central to ensuring trust between doctors and patients. The easiest ways to breach patient confidentiality are by casually discussing patients and by leaving medical records (paper or screen) where they can be seen, so always be on your guard.

You should be aware of principles of the Data Protection Act 1998†. The DOH has produced an NHS Code of Practice on confidentiality and NHS organisations have appointed Caldicott Guardians whose role is to protect patient information.

†See Chapter 9: Medical records and computers – Protecting patient information.

You must always obtain consent from the patient or someone authorised to act on their behalf before disclosing any medical information about them.

It is important to make it clear to a spouse, relatives and friends that you cannot discuss a patient's medical case without the patient's express consent‡. and you should reassure your patients of this. This may be particularly important to teenagers who may not see a GP if they have concerns about confidentiality.

‡See Chapter 13: Extras in the working day – Phone calls from concerned relatives.

If you do decide to disclose any information without a patient's consent then you must be prepared to explain why and justify your decision. Always seek medico-legal advice if you are unsure.

Disclosing medical information

Patients should understand that information about them will be shared amongst a team providing care for them. They should also be aware that information about them may be used for audit purposes. If a patient objects to the use of their information in this way then they should be made aware of the importance of sharing information, but ultimately their wishes should be respected. *Implied* consent is sufficient in these circumstances but other forms of disclosure require more *explicit* consent. Often disclosing information requires careful thought and judgement. Discuss cases with your colleagues or defence organisation if you are in doubt.

Disclosures to employers and insurance companies

GPs are regularly asked for information and to produce reports about their patients for third parties. Information can only be released with the patient's signed consent. Usually the third party sends the signed consent form to the GP together with the request for the report*.

*See *Chapter 12: Paperwork, certificates and benefits* – Other forms and certificates.

Patients can choose to see such reports before they are sent out, under the Access to Medical Reports Act 1988 (*Box 21.5*). As with accessing medical

---

Box 21.5   Access to Medical Reports Act 1988

- Allows patients to see reports written about them for employment or insurance purposes by doctors who are or have been responsible for their care
- Patients can apply to see the report *before* or *after* it is sent
- A copy of the report must be provided to the patient if requested and a 'reasonable fee' can be charged for this
- If the doctor is aware that the patient wants to see the report, he must not send it for 21 days allowing the patient time to access the report
- If the doctor knows the patient has seen the report, he must not send it until the patient confirms that it should be sent
- The doctor can amend the report if both doctor and patient agree about errors. Alternatively a patient statement can be added to the end of the document with their opinion on the disputed information.
- The patient can withdraw consent for a report to be sent after reading it
- A copy of the report must be kept by the doctor for 6 months from completion and the patient can access it until then

---

THE NEW GP SURVIVAL GUIDE

records* a GP can refuse the patient access to the report if they believe it would be likely to cause serious harm to the patient's physical or mental health.

*See Chapter 9: Medical records and computers – Patient access to medical records.

Disclosures required by law

Patients must be informed that information will be disclosed but their consent is not required, e.g. communicable disease reporting

Disclosures to court

If a judge or presiding officer of the court requests information about a patient then it can be disclosed. However, information requested by police or solicitors cannot be given without a patient's consent.

Disclosures to statutory regulatory bodies

If you have concerns about a colleague's performance in relation to particular patients, you must seek the patient's consent to disclose any identifiable information to the GMC or other body. If the patient withholds consent then the GMC will advise you what to do.

Disclosures in other circumstances

Before any disclosure, you need to carefully weigh up the benefits of disclosure against the harms of breaching confidentiality. Except in exceptional circumstances patients should always be asked for consent before releasing information. If a patient refuses to give consent, you can disclose information if you believe that the patient or a third party is being put at serious risk if you don't disclose. Be prepared to justify your decision.

Where a patient lacks the capacity to consent to disclosure of information, through immaturity, illness or mental incapacity, then try to persuade them to allow an appropriate person to be involved in the consultation. If this fails then act as above in their 'best interests'. Inform the patient beforehand that you are going to release information without their consent.

In cases of neglect, physical or sexual abuse, where the patient is unable to give or withhold consent, then information may be released to a statutory body or responsible person in order to prevent further harm to the patient.

After a patient's death

There remains an obligation to keep information confidential after a patient's death but this varies with circumstances. You should respect the patient's views on confidentiality if they were known to you prior to death. When information is requested you need to consider why the disclosure has been requested and carefully weigh up the benefits or harms of disclosure. You may need to discuss this with the patient's executor who should be fully informed of any disclosure. This is relevant where a life assurance company wishes to know the details of a patient's death before they agree to pay out. Again, seek advice.

COMPLAINTS

Complaints are unfortunately an almost inevitable part of practice. Mistakes will always be made, so be prepared to deal with their consequences. Clinical governance aims to reduce risk and provide a framework for managing mistakes when they occur, in a move towards a culture of openness.

In certain situations, a complaint may be anticipated and it is better to try to defuse the situation as it is occurring which may save a lot of time and worry later on. It may be better to involve other colleagues or the practice manager at an early stage, rather than waiting for a more formal complaint.

If you've made a mistake

If you know you've made a mistake then be honest about this, and discuss the matter with your colleagues or mentor or trainer. You may need to seek advice from your protection organisation. You must be open and honest with the patient, apologise, and make amends if necessary as soon as possible. It can be quite a relief to talk about a mistake you've made with your colleagues as you will usually find that you are not the only person to have ever made such an error.

Practice complaints procedure

All practices are required to have a documented complaints procedure and a nominated member of the practice, usually the manager, is responsible for dealing with complaints. When a patient wants to complain they should have the procedure explained and be offered written details on the complaints procedure. A patient may complain either verbally or in writing. They should have their complaint acknowledged within 2 working days and receive an explanation within 10 working days.

The NHS complaints procedure aims to resolve the majority of complaints at the 'local level' i.e. within the practice or PCO, if possible. Few complaints go beyond the practice complaints procedure, however, there are other agencies which can be involved if the patient is not satisfied (*Box 21.6*)*.

*See *Chapter 3: Working in the wider health service.*

Box 21.6   Agencies involved in complaints

PALS – Patient Advice and Liaison Service
- Available in every trust / PCO
- Provide advice and support for patients and families
- Liaise with other services to resolve problems
- Gateway to independent complaints procedures

PCO
- All PCOs must have a complaints manager
- Patients can complain to a PCO if they feel unable to complain to the practice
- PCOs provide support and advice for practices dealing with complaints

ICAS – Independent Complaints Advocacy Service
- Help individuals complain about NHS services

Healthcare Commission
- Deals with complaints not resolved at a local level
- Advises how best to proceed. May refer back to local organisations or set up a panel to investigate

Health Service Ombudsman
- Independent of NHS and government
- Patients can take their complaint to the ombudsman if not satisfied with the local or Healthcare Commission response

Patients may decide not to use the NHS complaints procedure but consult a lawyer directly instead, or do so having used the standard complaints procedure. Rarely the PCO may refer a case directly to the GMC or involve the police if serious professional misconduct or fraud is suspected. If a complaint is made against you and legal bells are sounding then contact your protection organisation immediately.

Dealing with a complaint against you

If you receive a complaint, discuss it with a partner, practice manager, mentor or trainer as soon as possible. Consider contacting your protection organisation depending on the nature of the complaint.

Review the medical records and write down anything further that you remember at this stage, for your own records. Don't be tempted to alter the records*. You may also need to write an official report.

Follow the practice complaints procedure and be prepared to meet the patient, perhaps with one of the partners and the practice manager. Listen to

*See *Chapter 9: Medical records and computers* – Amending medical records.

the patient, apologise if appropriate and provide reassurance that measures will be taken to avoid any mistake being repeated.

Even if the complaint is unfounded you should still allow the patient a chance to air their grievances and you may need to clear up any misunderstandings.

Complaints can be devastating for the individual doctor concerned. Expect to feel crestfallen, have a few sleepless nights and to find yourself being extra vigilant for a while afterwards. If a particular complaint causes ongoing worry for you seek support from medical colleagues and others early on, they should be able to help you to put the matter into perspective.

Learn what you can from a complaint; it does not necessarily mean you were in the wrong and need to change, but there is always something to review. It may be a source for a significant event analysis. Keep documentations of these for your appraisal and revalidation*.

*See *Chapter 20: Appraisal and revalidation.*

CLINICAL NEGLIGENCE

Negligence is a legal concept which implies that a reasonable standard of care was not achieved and that this is measured by a responsible body of professional opinion. It does not imply that the error was made on purpose or through active neglect.

In order for a negligence claim to be successful and damages paid all the following pre-requisites must be fulfilled:

1. The doctor owed a duty of care to the patient. You establish a duty of care whenever you enter into a therapeutic relationship with a patient.
2. The doctor was in breach of that duty.
3. The patient suffered harm.
4. That harm was caused by a breach of the duty of care (this can be hard to prove).

Damages (compensation) are payable to rectify the harm caused by the error. The amount is calculated to restore the claimant to the position they would have been in had the negligence not occurred.

Your protection organisation subscription should protect you against all the financial implications of such litigation. If negligence is clear and the defending doctor agrees that the patient suffered harm as a result of a breach in the duty of care then an out of court settlement is usually made.

SOURCES AND FURTHER READING

1. Knight B. *Legal Aspects of Medical Practice 5th Edition*. Churchill Livingstone. 1992.
2. Marquand P. *Introduction to Medical Law*. Butterworth Heinemann, 2000.
3. Medical Protection Society. *Common Problems: Managing the Risks in General Practice*. MPS, 2001.

4. RCGP / GPC. *Good Medical Practice for GPs.* Royal College of General Practitioners, 2002.

5. GMC, Guidance on Good Medical Practice booklet series:
   The Duties of a Doctor.
   Good Medical Practice, May 2001.
   Confidentiality: protecting and providing information, April 2004.
   Seeking Patients' Consent: the ethical considerations, November 1998.
   Intimate Examinations, December 2001.
   Serious Communicable Diseases, October 1997.
   Management in Health Care: the role of doctors, December 1999.
   Maintaining Good Medical Practice, July 1998.

6. NHS Executive. *Clinical Governance. Quality in the New NHS.* Department of Health, 1999.

7. Department of Health. *Good Practice in Consent Implementation Guide: consent to examination or treatment.* Department of Health, 2001.

8. Medical Protection Society. *Consent: A Complete Guide for GPs.* MPS, 2003.

9. BMA. *Access to Medical Reports Act (1988).* BMA, Dec 1988 (revised 1995).

10. Department of Health. *Confidentiality: NHS Code of Practice.* DOH, 2003.

11. Department of Health. *NHS Complaints Reform, Making Things Right.* DOH, 2003.

Chapter 22
Clinical issues with legal stipulations

INTRODUCTION

This chapter aims to clarify some clinical areas in which GPs have legal responsibilities.

ADVANCE DIRECTIVES

*See Chapter 21: Guidance for good professional practice – Competence.

Also known as advance statements, advance decisions and living wills, these written statements allow a legally competent* and adequately informed individual to let their wishes be known regarding treatment in the future, at a time when they may no longer be competent or be able to communicate. Patients may authorise or refuse specific treatments but they cannot legally request a specific treatment.

These statements are legally binding so long as the individual made the decision voluntarily and there is no reason to believe that they would have changed their mind in the time between making the statement and the relevant clinical situation arising.

GMC guidance states that when dealing with a patient who is not legally competent doctors should make efforts to find out if an advance directive exists and should abide by it if a specific clinical situation has occurred. Problems can arise if the directive doesn't apply specifically to the patient's current condition or the instructions are vague, in which case treatment should probably be given in the patient's best interests†.

†See Chapter 21: Guidance for good professional practice – Treating incompetent adults.

The onus for ensuring the advanced directive is drafted correctly lies with the patient. However, GPs may be asked by a patient to help draw up these documents or witness a patient's signature. A copy of an advance directive should be kept in the patient's medical record, which should be marked to this effect. The BMA suggests that patients should also carry a card indicating they have an advanced directive. Model advance directives are available from The Terrence Higgins Trust and the Voluntary Euthanasia Society (see *Sources and further reading*).

CHILD PROTECTION

> *If you suspect child abuse then document your concerns, seek the advice of health professional colleagues and report it to social services*

Child abuse may be physical, emotional and sexual and the term also includes neglect. Consider abuse where there is a vague story, odd parental behaviour, late presentation, failure to thrive, or unusual injuries. Abuse may come to light over time through the suspicions of all those involved in child care, including teachers. All areas have an Area Child Protection Committee

(ACPC) including social services, health professionals and the police, which is responsible for managing child abuse and producing local protocols. Familiarise yourself with the local protocols which should be available in your practice and be aware of who to call for advice and how to refer a child to social services (*Box 22.1*)*.

*See *Chapter 2: Working in the team.*

Box 22.1   Key players in Child Protection

Children and families social workers
- statutory duty to investigate cases of suspected abuse
- your first point of contact if you need to refer a case
- will check initially to see if a child is already known to them or on the Child Protection Register (see below)
- main role is to protect the child and support the family
- may contact you for medical information on a child reported to them by the school or even the police

Health visitors
- can follow up any low-grade suspicions and monitor children on the Child Protection Register
- involved in case conferences
- practice should have regular review meetings with them to discuss families of concern

Paediatricians and nurses
- Each trust must have a named doctor and named nurse (or midwife) who take the professional lead within the area for child protection issues
- responsible for dealing with suspected and confirmed abuse cases
- often involved in detailed sensitive examinations particularly where sexual abuse suspected
- should be available to discuss individual suspected cases with GPs

---

The Children Act 1989

> **Treat the child's interests as paramount**

This Act stipulates that the welfare and wishes of the child are paramount, particularly where court decisions are involved, and that children are to be kept informed and involved in decisions about their future. The law emphasises that the best way to protect that welfare is to support the care of children within their family unless this is not in their best interests. Removing a child from the family is not undertaken lightly. The Act highlights the need for the various agencies to co-operate in cases of child protection, and this has been reiterated by the Victoria Climbié inquiry.

Action in suspected abuse

You have a duty to act if you feel that a child has suffered significant harm or is likely to suffer significant harm. If a child is medically in need, due to serious injury or neglect, then refer them to hospital immediately. Make your suspicions of abuse explicit to the on-call paediatricians. You should then refer to social services unless the hospital is going to undertake this. Document fully your suspicions and details of the referral in the medical record.

In less acute cases follow your local protocols. Contact the duty social worker in the first instance. You or the social worker may involve a paediatrician for a further skilled assessment; be clear who is doing this. Even if the child is not seriously injured a brief hospital admission may be required for assessment and observation or to remove them from a dangerous situation. Any referral to social services can be done verbally but must be followed up in writing within 48 hours. Your referral should be acknowledged within one working day so if you have not heard back, contact them again.

It is good practice to discuss your concerns with your colleagues within the practice or a paediatrician or nurse with experience in child protection. You can do this without necessarily naming the child or the family.

Efforts should be made to keep the parents and child informed throughout. You should aim to get the consent of the child and their parents before any referral to social services or medical team unless you feel that seeking this consent would put the child at increased risk. Parents often feel very threatened at the prospect of social services involvement, so take the time to explain that you are making the referral to support the child and family, and that children are rarely removed from their homes. If the parents or the child refuse to allow you to involve social services, you can still make a referral if you feel that the child or another third party is at risk of serious harm. Discuss cases with your colleagues and medical protection organisation if these difficulties are arising. Keep meticulous notes about any child protection issue; include details about your concerns and any discussions or referrals.

Child protection investigations

Following a referral, social services will perform an initial assessment within 7 working days. If they feel that it is likely that significant harm had occurred or was likely to occur, section 47 enquires are then initiated which is a more detailed assessment. A child protection conference may then be organised if concerns are substantiated. If there are concerns that a crime has occurred, then the police will be involved.

Doctors have a duty to cooperate with child protection investigations. Consent should be obtained prior to disclosure of confidential information but not if this is contrary to the child's best interests, e.g. if the process of obtaining consent will put the child at increased risk or if it might prejudice a police investigation. Any disclosure of confidential information should be kept to a minimum, i.e. only information that is relevant to protect the safety of the child*.

*See *Chapter 21: Guidance on good professional practice –* Disclosing medical information.

Case conferences

Decisions about the child's future are often made by multidisciplinary case conferences. The conference should decide whether the child is at continuing risk of significant harm. GPs may be invited to attend these with members of the child protection team and other involved professionals, but they are often held during surgery time so it may be difficult to attend, in which case you may need to prepare a report. The outcomes of the conference may include:

- placement on to the Child Protection ('at risk') Register
- a Child Protection Plan for the future
- a 'Child in Need' plan may be drawn up for those not needing to go on the register but still requiring some input
- arrangements for review after an agreed period
- the need for a court order

Child Protection Register

These registers are kept by social services and hold information about children suffering or likely to suffer significant harm. Details of the type of abuse suffered, a personalised Child Protection Plan and names of key workers are included. The register has no legal standing but signifies both the level of concern and need for monitoring. Decisions to place the child on or remove the child's name from the register are made in case conferences and the GP and health visitors should be informed accordingly. Medical records should then be updated.

Emergency Protection Order

This court order allows a child to be removed from their normal residence or stipulates the circumstances under which a child can be seen, such as by a parent. Application for the order is usually made by social services. The order is effective immediately and without notice to the parent, lasts for 8 days, and can be extended for a further 7 days.

An exclusion requirement can be part of an emergency protection order. This can remove a perpetrator from the home rather than having to remove the child.

The police have separate powers to remove children to suitable accommodation when there is good reason to believe they may otherwise experience significant harm. Doctors may need police to invoke this power in order to admit a child to hospital where a child needs medical attention. The power lasts for 72 hours.

Other GP involvement in child protection

GPs have a vital role in supporting the children and family during and after investigations of abuse. Families may become divided both geographically and emotionally as a result of suspicions or revelations of abuse.

DEATHS

At the time of writing, the death certification system and Coroners Service were being reformed so expect some of this information to change.

Practical tips

- Accompany one of your colleagues when they are dealing with a death so you can learn about the process of confirmation of death, certification and liaison with the next of kin, funeral directors and coroner.
- Forewarn colleagues and the OOH service of any imminent expected deaths of patients under your care.
- When you are contacted to confirm an unexpected death of someone you don't know, ask for clinical details of the deceased and who will be there when you arrive. The police, as the coroner's representatives, will often be present at the scene.

Confirmation of death

Death can be confirmed by a doctor, some paramedics and some senior nurses. However, it is usually the GP who is called when the patient has died at home.

Perform your examination (*Box 22.2*); ask relatives if they would prefer to leave the room so you can do a full external inspection without feeling rushed or distressing them further. Look and feel for pacemakers in case a cremation certificate is required. Document your findings fully in the patient's medical record together with the time of your examination and the time of death if known (ask the relatives).

If you are working out of hours and the deceased is not a patient of yours or your practice then inform the family that they will need to contact the deceased's GP who may be able to issue the death certificate (see below). Let them know you will also contact the GP with all the necessary details.

Box 22.2   Confirmation of death

- No spontaneous respiration
- Pupils fixed and dilated
- No carotid pulse
- No heart or breath sounds over 1 minute
- Death confirmed at ....
- Time of death as reported to me ....

Remember to telephone or fax that GP, so they are aware of the situation before the family get in touch. OOH services may have a policy of reporting all OOH deaths to the coroner's officer who will then liaise with the patient's registered GP on the next working day.

Removal of the deceased

Plans for removal of the deceased depends on whether or not the coroner is involved.

If the coroner does not need to be informed then the body can be removed by a funeral director, usually available on-call 24 hours. The next of kin collects the death certificate from the patient's GP, takes it to the Registrar of Births, Deaths and Marriages who then issues the Order for Disposal required by the funeral director before burial or cremation can proceed.

If the coroner is informed, then the body must not be moved until there are specific instructions from the coroner's office. The coroner's officer may attend and arrange removal of the body (often to the local hospital mortuary). The coroner will decide if a post-mortem is needed and issue the death certificate after which the family can proceed with funeral arrangements.

Issuing the death certificate

A death certificate, a 'Medical Certificate of the Cause of Death', is usually completed by the patient's GP. To complete the certificate, you must know the cause of death and there must be no reason to inform the coroner. You do not have to see the body or have confirmed death (but should know who did). If you are unsure whether you can issue the certificate or not then discuss it with the coroner's officer; they are usually very helpful.

Your practice will have a book of death certificates with counterfoils. Complete these legibly and in full, avoiding vague causes of death such as 'old age'. You need only add your basic medical qualification to your signature, and put the surgery address under the 'your residence' section. Document the death certificate entry of 'cause of death' in the patient's medical records. You may need these details to complete a cremation form later.

Complete the certificate as soon as possible after the death out of courtesy to the relatives. Some religions have stipulations about burying the deceased within 24 hours of death so you may find yourself under some pressure to complete the certificate mid-surgery. Deaths in England and Wales must be registered within 5 days unless the coroner is involved and within 8 days in Scotland.

Informing the coroner

Some deaths (*Box 22.3*) must be reported to the coroner, via the coroner's office during working hours or via your local police station OOH. About one-third of deaths are reported, but not all will require a post-mortem.

If you do inform the coroner then always tell the relatives and the reasons why. Forewarn them that the coroner's officer may visit.

Box 22.3   Deaths to be reported to the coroner

- Cause of death unknown or uncertain
- Sudden or unexpected death
- Deceased not attended by a doctor in their last illness
- Deceased not seen by the doctor completing the death certificate after death or within 14 days before death
- Death whilst undergoing an operation or before recovery from anaesthetic
- Death linked to an abortion
- Death may be related to medical procedure or treatment or lack of medical care
- Death due to industrial disease
- There is a possibility of self-neglect or neglect by others
- Death occurred whilst in police custody
- The deceased was detained under the Mental Health Act
- Death due to poisoning including drugs and alcohol
- Unnatural deaths, deaths due to violence and accidents including: RTA, domestic accidents, falls, fires
- Criminal deaths: murder, manslaughter, infanticide, assisted suicide
- Suicides
- Infant deaths (including sudden infant deaths)

Cremation certificates

Only two of the eight forms for authorising cremation are relevant to GPs:

Form B

This is completed by the doctor who completed the death certificate. There is a statutory obligation to view the body after death so if you confirmed the death you can complete the form at the surgery. If you have not seen the deceased since they died you'll need to arrange with the funeral directors to view the body and complete the form there. Take the patient's medical records with you for reference. Remember to check for a pacemaker. The completion of the Cremation Form generates a fee. Unless the practice keeps th_____ cremation fees you receive for y_____

F____

T_____ ho has
b_____ tion of
t_____ ee and
c_____ s often
c_____ nother
c_____ en the
l

*See *Chapter 5: Contract and finances.*

East Kent Hospitals NHS Trust
LIBRARY REGISTRATION CARD

No.

LAST NAME
FIRST NAMES   Dr/Mr/Mrs/Miss/Ms
HOME ADDRESS: WORK ADDRESS:

POSTCODE:
TEL. No.::   POSITION:
EMAIL ADDRESS: TEL. No.::
                                                 BLEEP:

Leaving date/end of course (where applicable):

I agree to be responsible for all books borrowed by me or taken out in my name and I undertake to pay the cost of repair or replacement in respect of any damage or loss. The information provided will be held on a computer database and will only be used in relation to library business.

SIGNED:

DATE:

_____ lthough
_____ on their
_____ *le to the*
_____ *iver and*

_____ licences
_____ disabled,
_____ bled.

_____ g driving
_____ alth stipu-

GPs are involved in assessing fitness to drive for Group 2 licences and may be involved in confirming fitness in the over 70s for an ordinary licence. You may be required to provide a report and perform a medical examination for which a fee is payable.

Fitness to drive

Doctors have a duty to advise patients to notify the DVLA if they have a condition which affects their ability to drive.

However, it is the duty of the licence holder, and not the doctor, to inform the DVLA

Essentially anyone with a condition that might cause either a sudden or disabling event at the wheel, or affect the ability to control a vehicle safely, is not fit to drive. It is up to the DVLA to decide whether or not a patient is medically fit to drive so they need to be informed of relevant conditions. The '*At a Glance Guide*' is divided by medical condition for easy reference (*Box 22.4*) and you should familiarise yourself with the main stipulations.

You have a duty to ensure that your patient understands that their condition may impair their ability to drive and you should advise them that they are legally bound to inform the DVLA. If you forget to discuss it in the consultation then telephone or write to the patient, particularly if there is a new diagnosis.

Box 22.4   '*At a Glance Guide*': medical categories

	Important conditions included
Neurology	Epilepsy, stroke, brain tumours
Cardiovascular	Ischaemic heart disease, arrhythmias
Diabetes	
Psychiatry	Psychosis, dementia, depression
Drugs and alcohol misuse	
Visual problems	Visual acuity, visual field defects
Renal, respiratory and sleep disorders	Obstructive sleep apnoea
Miscellaneous	Elderly drivers

Following DVLA notification

Once the patient has notified the DVLA you may be contacted to provide a medical report. Use the guide to inform you as to whether you should advise the patient to abstain from driving pending the DVLA decision. Advise patients to inform their motor insurance company of any new illness as their insurance may be invalidated if they choose to ignore your advice.

For short periods of incapacity (i.e. up to 3 months), e.g. after surgery, drivers do not need to inform the DVLA but there are some neurological and cardiovascular exceptions to this. They will, however, need to inform their insurer.

Patients often react badly to being told that they may need to give up driving. They may even disagree with the diagnosis or its effect on driving. If this is the case then suggest a second opinion and advise them not to drive in the meantime.

Patients refusing to disclose to the DVLA

Very occasionally a patient will tell you outright that they have no intention of stopping driving or will continue to drive against your advice. In such difficult cases you may need to breach patient confidentiality in order to protect their safety and that of others. Follow the GMC guidance:

- If a patient is unable to understand that their condition affects their ability to drive (such as with dementia) then inform the DVLA immediately.
- If a patient continues to drive when unfit then persuade them to stop and this may include involving the next of kin (with the patients permission). If this is unsuccessful, or you are given evidence that they continue to drive, let the DVLA advisor know immediately.

If you do need to breach a patient's confidentiality, you must inform the patient before you do. You should also confirm that you have done so afterwards. Seek advice from your colleagues and medical defence organisation.

Seatbelts

The driver and all passengers must wear seatbelts but there are a few exceptions, e.g. patients with colostomies. 'Certificates of Exemption from Compulsory Seatbelt Wearing' are available from DOH and need to be signed by a doctor.

Alcohol and driving

The legal limit of blood alcohol is 50 mg/100 ml. There is great individual variation in alcohol metabolism so the oft-quoted statement that it takes 'one hour to clear a unit of alcohol' is not reliable.

THE MENTAL HEALTH ACT AND THE ACUTELY MENTALLY ILL PATIENT

Only a small proportion of mentally ill patients will ever need to be detained under the Mental Health Act. Relatively few of these will be for the first presentation of an acute psychosis. Sections can often be arranged over a period of days, as a situation deteriorates; the mental health team can be mobilised in advance and assessments made at a mutually convenient time. Although it may be quite evident that a section is required, in other less clear cut situations the decision will be shared between the GP, social worker and psychiatrist.

Go through some section papers before you need to use them in an emergency setting. Try and accompany one of your colleagues before you do your first section. Truly urgent sections always seem to crop up on busy days and can feel pretty chaotic but knowing who to contact and how can reduce the stress involved.

The Mental Health Act 1983 (England and Wales)

At the time of writing a new Mental Health Bill was going through parliament so be aware that this guidance may change. The DOH website contains information on the Act and how it affects health care professionals.

A patient with a mental disorder can be treated without their consent, i.e. compulsorily, for the mental disorder and any physical disorder arising from that mental disorder. There are specific grounds for admission (*Box 22.5*) under the Act. Scotland and Northern Ireland have their own legislation: Mental Health (Scotland) Act 1984 and the Mental Health (Northern Ireland) Order 1986 which are similar, but not identical.

Box 22.5 Grounds for admission under the Mental Health Act 1983 (England and Wales)

The patient suffers from a mental disorder of a nature or severity that justifies hospital admission
and
admission is in the interests of the patient's own health and safety and/or the safety of others
and
that voluntary admission is inappropriate – because the patient refuses admission or is unable to decide

---

Inclusions and exclusions of the Act

Mental disorder includes mental illness (which isn't actually defined in the Act), mental impairment (learning disability), psychopathic disorders and anorexia nervosa. It excludes drug and alcohol dependence, however, mental disorder can co-exist with, or arise from, drug and alcohol use or withdrawal.

Physical disorders where patients refuse consent to treatment cannot be treated under the Act, unless the physical disorder arises from the mental disorder. In such cases, if the patient lacks the capacity to decide then the 'best interests' principle should be used to determine if they should be treated*.

*See *Chapter 21: Guidance for good professional practice* – Treating incompetent adults.

Sections relevant to GPs

Only a few sections of the Act are relevant to GPs (*Box 22.6*). GPs should aim to use Section 2 or 3. The emergency Section 4 should be avoided unless there would be a dangerous delay in transferring the patient to hospital whilst a second medical opinion is awaited. Sections 2 and 4 are often converted to the longer Section 3 once the patient is admitted. You may be asked to attend a psychiatric ward to convert a patient to a more appropriate section.

Organising a section

GPs do not take overall responsibility for arranging an involuntary admission under the Mental Health Act but should work within the multi-disciplinary team which is usually led by the approved social worker or Section 12 approved doctor (see *Box 22.7*). CPNs do not have statutory involvement in sections but their input may inform your decision for an involuntary admission.

The request for a mental health assessment can come from a variety of sources:

- relatives, co-habitees and neighbours
- police or the ambulance service attending a violent patient
- ASW/CPN or other health professionals dealing with a patient

Only a social worker or nearest relative can actually apply for the section. The GP and psychiatrist then make the recommendation for a section.

Before you go

Liaise with the duty-approved social worker who should facilitate the section and arrange for the relevant professionals to be available. They may arrange to meet you at the patient's address or suitable place for assessment, e.g. the surgery. The ASW should bring the relevant paperwork.

Box 22.6　Mental Health Act 1983 (England and Wales) sections relevant to general practice

Section 2 'Admission for Assessment'
- Application by a social worker or nearest relative
- The applicant must have seen the patient within 14 days
- The patient can be admitted within 14 days of the application
- Requires medical recommendations from two doctors:
  - one Section 12 approved doctor (normally a psychiatrist)
  - one who knows the patient (usually the GP).
- Allows for admission to hospital for assessment for 28 days. Treatment can also be given
- Patient can appeal within the first 14 days

Section 3 ' Admission for Treatment'
- Application, assessment and recommendation as for Section 2
- Diagnosis must be known
- Admission up to 6 months and renewable
- Patient can appeal during first 6 months

Section 4 'Admission in an Emergency'
- Application by social worker or nearest relative
- Application valid for 24 hours
- Requires only one medical recommendation: either a doctor with prior knowledge of the patient, e.g. the GP or approved doctor
- Allows for admission for assessment for 72 hours only
- Patient should be admitted within 24 hours of the application or medical recommendation
- Should be reserved for 'emergency' situations when organising a Section 2 would cause unnecessary delay
- Patient cannot appeal

Once there

You need to:

- put your own safety first
- assess the patient and decide if hospital admission is needed
- try to persuade the patient to agree to voluntary admission if possible
- where they refuse, establish whether there are grounds for involuntary admission under the Mental Health Act

---

Box 22.7   Key players in mental health assessments

Approved Social Worker (ASW)
- key to the whole process
- may know the patient already
- will have the relevant section papers
- will do their own mental health assessment (MHA) on the patient
- will find the Section 12 psychiatrist (below) for the assessment
- have a statutory duty to inform the patient's family of the section
- may be able to locate a bed for the patient
- keep their contact number in your on-call paperwork

Section 12 approved doctor
- usually a psychiatrist
- will often be the Responsible Medical Officer (RMO) taking overall responsibility for the section
- available on-call in the community
- assess patients to determine the need for a section in addition to the GP's opinion
- receive a fee for this service
- contactable via the approved social worker (ASW)

After the assessment

Once you have made your assessment and recommended a section, then complete and sign the papers and leave them with the social worker. Unless the patient needs acute medical treatment, such as sedation, you can then go. Document fully your assessment and reasoning for use of the Mental Health Act in the medical record.

If a section is not needed

Arrange alternative management such as medication, voluntary admission or outpatient review with increased input from the CMHT in the meantime.

Appeals against sections

Patients and nearest relatives can appeal to have sections revoked by application to a Mental Health Review Tribunal which consists of a psychiatrist, lawyer and a lay member. The Mental Health Act Commission, a special health authority which oversees the operation of the Mental Health Act, also investigates complaints made by detained patients.

Discharge

The hospital should always let you know directly when a patient admitted involuntarily is discharged. A formal multidisciplinary assessment is arranged under the Care Programme Approach and details the professionals involved; treatment and dates for review team meetings should be forwarded on to you. A key worker is allocated to coordinate the care plan and ensure communication between professionals.

NOTIFIABLE DISEASES

Under the Public Health (Control of Disease) Act 1984 and Public Health (Infectious Diseases) Regulations 1988, doctors are obliged to notify the 'relevant local authority officer' of the identity and address of any person suspected of having a notifiable disease (*Box 22.8*) or food poisoning. If in doubt discuss the case with your local Public Health Department.

In general practice, you are most likely to make notifications for food poisoning and hepatitis. Microbiology labs will often prompt you to notify by a comment on the pathology report.

Your practice will have a book of notification forms for completion together with the local forwarding address to the Medical Officer for Environmental Health. A small fee is payable. Always inform any patients

---

Box 22.8   Notifiable diseases

Acute encephalitis	Paratyphoid fever
Acute poliomyelitis	Plague
Anthrax	Rabies
Cholera	Relapsing fever
Diphtheria	Rubella
Dysentery	Scarlet fever
Food poisoning	Smallpox
Leptospirosis	Tetanus
Leprosy	Tuberculosis
Malaria	Typhoid fever
Measles	Typhus fever
Meningitis	Viral haemorrhagic fever
Meningococcal septicaemia	Viral hepatitis
Mumps	Whooping cough
Ophthalmia neonatorum	Yellow fever

Reproduced from the Public Health Act 1988.

you notify, explain why and warn them that they may be contacted by Public Health Department staff, particularly if they are food-handlers.

POWER OF ATTORNEY

This legal document allows someone to give control of their financial affairs and property to another (the attorney). This is particularly relevant in the management of patients with dementia.

Ordinary power of attorney is appropriate where someone needs another person to manage their affairs temporarily but is invalidated if the donor becomes mentally incapacitated, i.e. legally incompetent. An enduring power of attorney continues even if the donor becomes mentally incapacitated. It is important to consider this in the early stages of dementia as the donor must have sufficient competence to grant the power in the first place. The Mental Capacity Bill which is before Parliament at the time of writing will create a lasting power of attorney. Appointed attorneys will be able to make financial, health and personal welfare decisions on behalf of a patient should they later become incapacitated.

GPs may be asked to comment on a patient's capacity to agree to setting up a power of attorney, but it may be prudent to get another specialist opinion, e.g. from a psychogeriatrician. There are specific guidelines on assessing mental capacity from the BMA in conjunction with the Law Society (see *Sources and further reading*).

Advise anyone applying for power of attorney (usually a relative), to contact a citizens advice bureau, solicitor or law centre to ensure all the legal requirements are met.

TERMINATION OF PREGNANCY

The GP is often the first place a woman will go when she wants a termination of pregnancy (TOP). If you have conscientious or religious objections you are not obliged to advise, refer or sign the paperwork for TOPs. You do, however, have a duty to refer your patient promptly to another doctor who is willing to counsel and refer as needed, which will usually be one of your GP colleagues.

The Abortion Act 1967 and the Human Fertilisation and Embryology Act 1990

These Acts allow a TOP to be carried out legally in the circumstances specified on an HSA1 form, 'Certificate A' (*Box 22.9*).

A termination can be carried out at any gestation if there is a substantial risk that the child would be seriously handicapped or the mother's life or health is in grave danger. Other criteria allow for a termination up to the end of the 24th week of pregnancy. Most requests for terminations in general practice will be satisfied by the criteria in C.

The HSA1 form must be completed and signed by two doctors who have seen the woman but it is not necessary for both to examine the woman. The GP is usually the first signatory and the form is then sent with the referral to the TOP clinic for the clinic or hospital doctor to complete it.

A further form is sent to the Chief Medical Officer (CMO) by the doctor undertaking the procedure within 14 days, confirming that the termination has been carried out.

All terminations must be carried out in approved hospitals, which include some private clinics. Most regions offer an NHS-based termination service through the hospital or community gynaecology service but this may be contracted out to a local private or voluntary sector service.

Arranging NHS terminations

Find out how best to refer locally and what different clinics will offer, e.g. medical and late terminations. In some regions women may arrange a clinic appointment themselves through a central booking service but they may still require a GP referral letter. Have this number to hand in your surgery. Otherwise your practice secretary or receptionist should arrange the appointment by telephone and the woman should be advised to return to collect their referral letter, HSA1 form and appointment time.

Advise women they will not have the actual termination on the day of their clinic appointment.

Where dates are uncertain or the woman presents late you may wish to arrange an urgent dating ultrasound, or refer them urgently so the clinic can do this.

Private clinics

Several private and voluntary sector agencies offer pregnancy counselling and terminations. Charges are around £350–600 and women may self refer. This may be an option for those who can afford it and find the NHS wait too long.

Well-known organisations include the British Pregnancy Advisory Service and Marie Stopes Clinics (see *Sources and further reading*)

SOURCES AND FURTHER READING

General

1. Knight B. *Legal Aspects of Medical Practice, 5th edition.* Churchill Livingstone, 1992.
2. Marquand P. *Introduction to Medical Law.* Butterworth Heinemann, 2000.

Advance directives

3. British Medical Association. *Code of Practice and Guidance on Advance Statements.* BMA, 1995.
4. Panting G. How does a living will affect the care you give your patient? *Guidelines in Practice*, **7**: October 2004.
5. The Terrence Higgins Trust, 52–54 Grays Inn Road, London WC1X 8JU, Tel: 0845 122 1200, www.tht.org.uk
6. Voluntary Euthanasia Society, 13 Prince of Wales Terrace, London W8 5PG, Tel: 020 7937 7770, www.ves.org.uk

Child protection

7. British Medical Association. *Doctors Responsibilities in Child Protection Cases.* BMA, 2004.

8. Department of Health. *What to Do if You're Worried a Child is Being Abused.* DOH, 2003.
9. National Society for the Prevention of Cruelty to Children, www.nspcc.org.uk

Deaths

10. Death and Cremation Certificates.
11. Department of Work and Pensions. *D49: What to do after a death in England and Wales.* DWP, 2003.

Driving

12. Driver and Vehicle Licensing Agency (DVLA), www.dvla.gov.uk
13. Driver and Vehicle Licensing Agency. *At a Glance Guide to the Current Medical Standards of Fitness to Drive.* DVLA, Sept 2004.
14. General Medical Council. *Confidentiality: Protecting and Providing Information.* GMC, 2004.

Mental Health

15. Bradley J.J. *The Mental Health Act 1983 (England and Wales), Mental Health (Patients in the Community) Act 1995.* Medical Protection Society, 1997.
16. Department of Health. *Improving Mental Health Law. Towards a New Mental Health Act.* DOH, 2004.
17. Department of Health, www.dh.gov.uk

Notifiable diseases

18, Notification certificates.
19. Health Protection Agency, www.hpa.org.uk

Power of attorney

20. BMA and The Law Society. *Assessment of Mental Capacity: Guidance for Doctors and Lawyers.* 1995.

Termination of pregnancy

21. British Medical Association. *The Law and Ethics of Abortion. BMA Views.* BMA, 1999.
22. British Pregnancy Advisory Service, www.bpas.org.uk
23. Marie Stopes International, www.mariestopes.org.uk

Chapter 23
Career options for general practitioners

INTRODUCTION

There are numerous opportunities in general practice. The traditional model of working as a partner within a practice still offers many benefits but GPs are now able to choose alternative working patterns. GPs are in a great position to work flexibly, in different posts with control over their hours and conditions. GPs can combine their interests to create a 'portfolio career'*.

*See *Chapter 1: Working in general practice*, for a description of the various types of GP.

The term non-principal and sessional GP can be used interchangeably.

WORKING AS A SESSIONAL GP

Getting started

Sessional GPs must be on a 'Performers List' in order to work in general practice in a given area. Contact the local PCO for details of how to apply. There are many local groups for non-principals which are set up to share ideas, job information and keep up to date with clinical issues. You should also consider joining the The National Association of Sessional GPs (NASGP). Their website provides lots of useful information and includes a list of local groups.

Locums

Working as a GP locum is an excellent way to work flexibly and see how other practices operate. Working in different settings can give you clear ideas about what you want when, and if, you commit to a permanent post.

Before starting work as a locum:

- You need to have all your own equipment so re-stock your bag. You may have to buy your drug supplies on a private prescription.
- Inform your medical protection organisation of your intention to work as a locum.
- Ensure GMC subscriptions are up to date.
- Have confirmation of your hepatitis B immune status.
- Make photocopies of your current GMC certificate, medical protection certificate and JCPTGP certificate (or PMETB equivalent) and provide the practices with these.
- Ensure you have a mobile phone, email address and diary and devise a system to avoid double booking.
- Have two recent references. Practices may start asking for these as it is the responsibility of the practice to ensure you are up to the job.

Box 23.1   Finding locum work

- Get a list of all local practices from the PCO
- Update your CV and circulate it to local practices with a covering letter to the practice manager
- Let your training practice know you are looking for work
- Ask your VTS colleagues to inform you of any work in their practice
- Register with local locum groups or agencies (see *BMJ* and GP press)
- Put up a notice at the OOH service if they are agreeable
- Look for adverts in the *BMJ Classified* and the GP press
- Contact hospital personnel departments if you would consider some hospital locums

---

Money matters

Locums are self-employed (see *Box 23.2*) and you will need to register as such by informing the Inland Revenue. They will provide you with information about registering to pay class 2 (self-employed) National Insurance contributions. You will be responsible for paying your own tax and you will need to keep money aside for this (approximately one-third of your income). It may be wise to discuss your financial status with a small business advisor at your bank and an accountant. The Association of Independent Specialist Medical Accountants (AISMA) can put you in contact with an accountant in your area.

Box 23.2   Useful contacts for locums

Helpline for the Newly Self Employed 0845 915 4515
Register you as self employed and provide some information on tax and national insurance
Self Assessment Helpline 0845 900 0444
Advise about queries on tax returns
www.inlandrevenue.gov.uk
NHS Pensions Agency 01253 774 967
www.nhspa.gov.uk

You can claim work-related expenses against tax (subscriptions, medical protection costs, telephone, stationery, travel expenses, etc.) so keep all receipts. Consider keeping a spreadsheet of your income and outgoings as you go. It's a good idea to have a separate bank account or credit card for work-related costs.

Confirm or negotiate fees before you commit to a locum and establish whether you will be paid an hourly, sessional or all-day rate. You should decide whether you are prepared to do visits, sign repeat prescriptions and be on-call and whether these are included in your rate. Always confirm in writing what you have agreed to do.

It may be difficult to know at what level to set your rates. The local market forces will dictate what you can charge. Have a chat with other locums or practice managers to get a ball park figure of average rates. *Medeconomics* publishes a survey of locum earnings which will give you an idea of the range of charges in your area. You will miss out on holiday, sick and maternity pay and you will not have paid study leave so take this into account when deciding how much you charge and how much you need to work and earn.

You will need to devise a system of producing invoices and receipts. Invoice practices at the time of the session or soon afterwards and keep a record of unpaid sessions so you can remind practice managers.

Your income may be irregular so you may need a 'cushion' or reasonable overdraft facility to ensure your regular bills are covered. It may be wise to have the equivalent of at least 3 months earnings saved in case you are unable to work. It is particularly important for locums to have arranged income protection as they will not be entitled to the benefits that employees can expect.

NHS locums are entitled to contribute to the NHS pension scheme, so keep accurate details of your locum earnings, who you worked for and when. You will have to send off forms on a monthly basis which need to be signed by the practice managers*.

*See *Chapter 5 Contract and finances* - Pensions.

Support

It is common to feel under-confident when starting out so work in larger practices initially and avoid isolated single-handed practices. Confirm that other doctors will be working at the same time and don't hesitate to ask for clinical advice.

Practices should provide you with a locum pack including the main paperwork you need, practice telephone numbers, prescribing policy and referral information. Avoid practices with unfamiliar computer systems.

You should also negotiate the length of surgeries, consultation time and breaks you require before undertaking the locum. Do not agree to do visits, telephone consultations, on-call or sign repeat prescriptions unless you feel comfortable. Most practices are flexible about this.

Salaried GPs

PCOs, PMS and GMS practices and alternative providers of medical services (APMS) offer a number of different types of salaried and assistant posts. Retainers, returners and flexible careers scheme GPs are also salaried but the schemes are targeted at specific groups.

Salaried schemes may offer clinical sessions in a practice with sessions in another specialty or research. These posts can be ideal for newly qualified GPs and may include protected time for peer support, audit and practice development. However, there is a great variety of posts and not all have the same benefits so search carefully for a post which suits your needs and interests.

As part of the nGMS contract, the BMA has produced model terms and conditions for salaried GPs working in a GMS practice and for GPs employed by a PCO. There are also model contracts for GPs on the flexible careers scheme and retainer scheme. This should mean that salaried doctors are employed under similar terms and conditions throughout the country. The specifications regarding maternity leave, study leave and sick leave are very favourable compared with contracts that many salaried GPs have been employed under in the past. You should make sure that you are employed under terms and conditions as specified in one of these model contracts. All GMS practices are required to offer terms and conditions that are no less favourable than the model in the nGMS contract. The BMA advises that salaried GPs employed by other practices are also employed under these terms and conditions*.

*See also *Chapter 5: Contract and finances.*

Salaries vary around the country, however, the Doctors and Dentists Review Body has advised on the appropriate range of salary for a salaried GP and the BMA has produced guidance on how to negotiate salaries.

Check the *BMJ Classified* for adverts and contact you local PCO about salaried GP schemes in your area.

Retainer scheme

This scheme provides GPs who have outside commitments, which prevent them from working full time, with the opportunity to work regularly on a part-time basis, retain their skills and keep up to date. Retainers are employed by a practice to work between one and four sessions a week for up to five years. For short periods it is possible to work more sessions than this with the agreement of the deanery. Retainers are committed to attend a certain number of educational sessions a year. The BMA has produced a model contract for retainers.

Women with young families are the main group who are employed via the retainer scheme. The practice is reimbursed part of the retainer's salary and the retainer will also receive a contribution from the deanery for professional expenses. The retainer must justify why they can only work a few sessions a week and have long-term plans to return to general practice more fully in the future.

Returner scheme

This scheme is aimed at GPs who are currently not working or not working within general practice and GPs who are exclusively doing locum work. The scheme was set up to encourage these GPs to return to general practice in a substantive post. After undergoing an individual learning-needs assessment, the GP undergoes a period of refresher training and assessment which is normally between 6 and 12 months. The returner is normally placed in a training practice for which the practice receives a training grant. The training is planned with a 'return co-ordinator' from the postgraduate deanery.

GPs applying for the scheme should have the intention to take up a substantive general practice post for a minimum of 2 years.

There is a returners hotline for interested GPs: 0845 606 0345.

Flexible careers scheme

This is open to GPs who want greater choices about how and when they work. It is aimed at GPs who want to work less than 50% of full time and want to work in a flexible way or have a portfolio career. It may also be suitable for those nearing retirement or those wishing to return after retiring.

GPs can work between two and five sessions a week but sessions can be annualized. This enables GPs to organize their sessions to fit in with other commitments, e.g. school holidays. Flexible careers scheme doctors are able to work some locum sessions.

There is a model contract produced by the BMA. The scheme lasts for up to 3 years but the GP must have a planned exit strategy when entering the scheme. The employer receives reimbursement for part of the flexible careers scheme doctor's salary and the GP will receive a contribution towards professional expenses.

PARTNERSHIP

Many GPs still see partnership as the ultimate goal but deciding when and where can be problematic. It is increasingly common for GPs to move around and change partnerships so it need not be viewed as a lifelong commitment.

Getting to know patients, families and communities long term can be very rewarding. Deciding how you work and developing your practice and services can be very stimulating. There is also the benefit of permanence, job security and usually increased income.

Doing your research

Choosing a partnership is a complicated business (*Box 23.3*), so take your time to research it fully. Individuals will have different lists of priorities. Things to take into consideration are the location and population of the practice. You will need to know the list size and the number of whole time equivalents working within the practice. Take into account the staff, building and facilities within the practice. You should know how work is distributed, e.g. on-calls, visits, length of surgeries, and whether there is flexibility in the system. Doctors may have specialist interests which may be beneficial for the practice but a new partner may be expected to develop a role. You will need to negotiate any regular half days or days off and find out whether this is compatible with the practice.

Before agreeing to a position, spend time with each partner and the practice manager, and ask the opinion of other local doctors. Time spent as a locum is an excellent way to see the day-to-day running of the practice. If you are keen on a place but not absolutely sure then ask to work for 6–12 months in a salaried capacity before you commit more fully. Otherwise consider an opt-out clause in your agreement after 3–6 months of working as a partner. No practice is perfect but it's better to know the personalities and potential problems before you start.

Financial matters

You must know what the situation is regarding remuneration. Ask to see the practice accounts and practice agreement; it may be helpful to go through these with a member of the practice. The GPC has produced guidance about what should be included in a partnership agreement and the BMA can provide advice to members. GPs entering into an agreement should also seek financial and legal advice.

Remember principals are self-employed and their income is generated by the business work of the practice. How they divide it between partners is another matter.

With recruitment difficulties in many parts of the UK a new partner is often in an excellent position to negotiate full parity and a delay before contributing to practice assets.

Salaried partners

These increasingly prevalent posts are a good option for doctors who want security and permanence without all the management and financial commitments of full partnership. There is an obvious overlap between such posts and salaried GPs.

CLINICAL SESSIONAL WORK

There are many opportunities to work as a GP on a sessional basis for NHS and other organizations (*Box 23.4*). This can be on a regular or *ad hoc* basis. Posts may be advertised in the *BMJ*, otherwise ask around locally or contact the organizations themselves. You may need some prior experience of the specialty depending on the post applied for.

Box 23.4   Opportunities for sessional work

NHS
- Out of hours services
- Family planning
- Pregnancy advisory services
- Genitourinary medicine
- Homeless projects
- Drug and alcohol services
- NHS Walk-In centres
- Clinical assistant in hospital outpatients

Private
- Private screening medicals, e.g. BUPA
- Drug rehabilitation units
- Medical support for events
- Private general practice

GPS WITH A SPECIALIST INTEREST

With the intention of increasing the number of outpatient appointments happening in the community and with the development of enhanced services, more GPs are working as GPwSI*.

*See Chapter 1: Working in General Practice – GP contract.

Seeing a GPwSI has the advantages of reducing waiting times, improving convenience for patients and encouraging GPs to enhance their careers by developing or pursuing an interest.

Posts for GPwSI are developed locally according to the specific needs of the population and the skills available amongst general practitioners. The DOH and RCGP have produced some guidelines on the roles of GPwSIs and how evidence of a specialist interest may be established. Clinical areas covered in the guidance include care of older people, child protection, dermatology, diabetes, drug misuse, echocardiography, emergency care, ENT, headaches, mental health, musculoskeletal conditions, palliative care, and sexual health.

If you are interested in becoming a GPwSI you should liaise with your PCO about current and future opportunities and look at the guidelines on the DOH website.

ACADEMIC POSTS

Primary care is a growing academic discipline and there are often full or part-time lecturer, researcher and other posts available at your local academic department of general practice or primary care.

Funding is available for individual research work from various sources. Research general practices exist around the country with special funding.

Working for a higher degree (MSc or PhD) in primary care will provide a good basis for full time academia or continuing with sessional research work throughout your clinical career.

EDUCATION

Numerous opportunities exist for GPs to get involved in medical education.

A considerable proportion of undergraduate student teaching is now undertaken in general practice.

Pre-registration doctors are due to spend training time in general practice as part of Modernising Medical Careers, providing a new education role for GPs.

General practice trainers need to have been working in general practice for at least 3 years, have the MRCGP exam and undergone some training. The practice needs to be accredited and the trainer needs to undergo regular assessment and re-approval. Course organizing and working for the postgraduate deanery are other job opportunities with an educational focus.

POLITICS AND MANAGEMENT

Representing general practitioners at local or national level appeals to many GPs*.

*See *Chapter 3: Working in the wider health service.*

A wide variety of opportunities exist for GPs within their local PCO. Having an influence on local policies and procedures may provide stimulating sessional work for some. The posts generally cover your locum costs or loss of income costs and may contribute towards childcare.

OTHER CAREERS AND QUALIFICATIONS

General practice is an ideal starting point for many other careers, e.g. public health, sports medicine, medical journalism, and occupational medicine. There are many postgraduate diplomas and other qualifications that are open to you as a GP. These qualifications may simply allow you to pursue an interest or they may help you in developing your career within general practice or an alternative specialty.

WORKING ABROAD

The *BMJ Careers* section carries advertised posts for GPs to work abroad. Australia and New Zealand have posts available, usually in areas where they have found difficulty recruiting.

Voluntary organizations such as Voluntary Services Overseas (VSO), International Health Exchange, Médecins sans Frontières and Merlin have some placements in developing countries or war-torn areas. They may require a relatively long-term commitment. Working as a ship's doctor is another option provided you have sea legs!

SOURCES AND FURTHER READING

1. Aquino P., Jones P. (eds) *Career Options in General Practice.* Radcliffe Medical Press, 2004.
2. National Association of Sessional GPs, www.nasgp.org.uk
3. Inland Revenue, www.inlandrevenue.gov.uk
4. NHS Pensions Agency, www.nhspa.gov.uk
5. Coull R. *Locum Doctor Survival Guide,* www.locum123.com
6. Association of Medical Accountants, www.aisma.org.uk
7. General Practitioners Committee. *The New GMS Contract Explained – Focus on Salaried GPs.* BMA, 2004.
8. BMA. *Guidance for Salaried GPs: Negotiating your salary.* BMA, 2003 (updated 2004).
9. General Practitioners Committee. *Partnership Agreements Guidance.* BMA, 2004.
10. BMA, www.bma.org.uk
11. London Deanery Sessional GPs Survival Handbook, www.londondeanery.ac.uk
12. Department of Health. www.dh.gov.uk, provides information on GPwSI.
13. Voluntary Service Overseas, www.vso.org.uk
14. International Health Exchange, www.ihe.org.uk
15. Médecins sans Frontières, www.msf.org
16. Merlin, www.merlin.org.uk

Appendix 1
Useful websites

General professional

General Medical Council, www.gmc-uk.org
British Medical Association, www.bma.org.uk
Royal College of General Practitioners, www.rcgp.org.uk
Royal Society of Medicine, www.rsm.ac.uk
Medical Protection Society, www.mps.org.uk
Medical Defence Union, www.the-mdu.com
National Association of Sessional GPs, www.nasgp.org.uk

Organisations related to GP training and appraisal

National Office for Summative Assessment, www.nosa.org.uk
Joint Committee on Postgraduate Training for General Practice,
    www.jcptgp.org.uk
List of UK deaneries, www.nosa.org.uk/contacts/deaneries.htm
Postgraduate Medical Education and Training Board, www.pmetb.org.uk
Appraisal and revalidation, www.revalidationuk.info,
    www.appraisals.nhs.uk

Heath service and related organisations

National Health Service, www.nhs.uk
Department of Health, www.dh.gov.uk.
NHS Scotland, www.show.scot.nhs.uk
Department of Health, Social Services and Public Safety in Northern
    Ireland, www.dhsspsni.gov.uk
Health of Wales Information Service, www.wales.nhs.uk
Choose and Book, www.chooseandbook.nhs.uk
Department for Work and Pensions Corporate Medical Group website,
    www.dwp.gov.uk/medical
Healthcare Commission, www.chai.org.uk
Health Protection Agency, www.hpa.org.uk
London Ambulance Service, www.londonambulance.nhs.uk

National Clinical Assessment Authority, www.ncaa.nhs.uk
National Patient Safety Agency, www.npsa.nhs.uk
National Primary Care Development Team, www.npdt.org
National Programme for Information Technology in the NHS,
    www.npfit.nhs.uk
NHS Cancer Screening Programmes, www.cancerscreening.nhs.uk
NHS Confederation, www.nhsconfed.webhoster.co.uk
NHS Information Authority, www.nhsia.nhs.uk
NHS University, www.nhsu.nhs.uk
World Organisation of Family Doctors, www.globalfamilydoctor.com

Financial

Association of Independent Specialist Medical Accountants,
    www.aisma.org.uk
Inland Revenue, www.inlandrevenue.gov.uk
Medeconomics, www.medeconomics.co.uk
NHS Pensions Agency, www.nhspa.gov.uk
Office for Manpower Economics, www.ome.uk.com

Royal Colleges, faculties and professional associations

British Association of Dermatologists, www.bad.org.uk
British Hypertension Society, www.bhsoc.org
British Society of Gastroenterology, www.bsg.org.uk
British Thoracic Society, www.brit-thoracic.org.uk
Faculty of Family Planning and Reproductive Healthcare,
    www.ffprhc.org.uk
Faculty of Pharmaceutical Medicine, www.fpm.org.uk
Faculty of Public Health Medicine, www.fph.org.uk
The Renal Association, www.renal.org
Royal College of Obstetricians and Gynaecologists, www.rcog.org.uk
Royal College of Paediatrics and Child Health, www.rcpch.ac.uk
Royal College of Physicians, www.rcplondon.ac.uk
Royal College of Psychiatrists, www.rcpsych.ac.uk
Royal Colleges of Ophthalmologists, www.rcophth.ac.uk

Prescribing

British National Formulary, www.bnf.org
Medicines and Healthcare Products Regulatory Agency, www.mhra.gov.uk
National Prescribing Centre, www.npc.co.uk
Prescription Pricing Authority, www.ppa.org.uk
No free lunch, www.nofreelunch-uk.org

Sources of clinical information for doctors

National Electronic Library for Health – provides access to a large number
of specialist libraries, guidelines and databases. The Cochrane database,
Clinical Evidence, *Drugs and Therapeutics Bulletin* and *Bandolier* can be
accessed via this site, www.nelh.nhs.uk
National Library for Health, www.library.nhs.uk
Bandolier, www.jr2.ox.ac.uk/bandolier
British Medical Journal, www.bmj.com
Clinical Evidence, www.clinicalevidence.com
DoctorOnline, www.doctoronline.nhs.uk
eGuidelines, www.eguidelines.co.uk
GP Online, www.gponline.com
General Practice Notebook, www.gpnotebook.co.uk
National Institute for Clinical Excellence, www.nice.org.uk
Prodigy, www.prodigy.nhs.uk
Scottish Intercollegiate Guidelines Network, www.sign.ac.uk

Organisations with an educational focus

MRCGP exam, www.mrcgpexam.co.uk
BMJ Learning, www.bmjlearning.com
JointZone, www.jointzone.org.uk

Working overseas

Voluntary Service Overseas, www.vso.org.uk
International Health Exchange, www.ihe.org.uk
Médecins sans Frontières, www.msf.org
Merlin, www.merlin.org.uk

Other useful websites for doctors

Doctors.net, www.doctors.net.uk
onmedica.net, www.onmedica.net
BMJ Bookshop, www.bmjbookshop.com
BMJ Careers, www.bmjcareers.com
Locum doctors website, www.locum123.com

Patient orientated sites

Patient UK, www.patient.co.uk
BestTreatments, www.besttreatments.co.uk
NHS Direct Online, www.nhsdirect.nhs.uk
Patients Association, www.patients-association.com
Citizens Advice Bureau, www.citizensadvice.org.uk

Medic Alert, www.medicalert.org.uk
Driver and Vehicle Licensing Agency, www.dvla.gov.uk
DIPEx, www.dipex.org

Clinical topics

These sites may be useful to you or your patients

Adolescent health	Teenage Health Freak, www.teenagehealthfreak.org
Cancer	Macmillan Cancer Relief, www.macmillan.org.uk
	CancerBACUP, www.cancerbacup.org.uk
Cardiology	British Heart Foundation, www.bhf.org.uk
Child health	National Society for the Prevention of Cruelty to Children, www.nspcc.org.uk
Dermatology	Acne Support Group, www.stopspots.org
	National Eczema Society, www.eczema.org
Diabetes	Diabetes UK, www.diabetes.org.uk
Diet/obesity	The British Nutrition Foundation, www.nutrition.org.uk
	National Obesity Forum, www.nationalobesityforum.org.uk
Drug /alcohol abuse	Alcohol Concern, www.alcoholconcern.org.uk
	Alcoholics Anonymous, www.alcoholics-anonymous.org.uk
	Talk to Frank (drug information), www.talktofrank.com
Elderly care	Age Concern, www.ageconcern.org.uk
Gastroenterology	Irritable Bowel Syndrome Network, www.ibsnetwork.org.uk
Infections	Terrence Higgins Trust (HIV information), www.tht.org.uk
Men's health	Men's Health Forum, www.menshealthforum.org.uk
Mental health	Depression Alliance, www.depressionalliance.org
	The Mental Health Foundation, www.mentalhealth.org.uk
	Mind, www.mind.org.uk
Musculoskeletal	National Osteoporosis Society, www.nos.org.uk
	Arthritis Research Campaign, www.arc.org.uk
Neurology	The Stroke Association, www.stroke.org.uk
	Meningitis Trust, www.meningitis-trust.org.uk
	Alzheimer's Society, www.alzheimers.org.uk
	Epilepsy Action, www.epilepsy.org.uk
	Multiple Sclerosis Society, www.mssociety.org.uk
	Parkinson's Disease Society, www.parkinsons.org.uk
	Migraine Trust, www.migrainetrust.org
	National Autistic Society, www.nas.org.uk
Palliative care	Marie Curie Cancer Care, www.mariecurie.org.uk

	Hospice information, www.hospiceinformation.info
Renal	UK National Kidney Federation, ww.kidney.org.uk
Respiratory	Asthma UK, www.asthma.org.uk
Smoking	Giving Up Smoking (NHS), www.givingupsmoking.co.uk
Women's health	National Childbirth Trust, www.nctpregnancyandbabycare.com
	BladderZone, www.bladderzone.co.uk
	FPA (formerly the Family Planning Association), www.fpa.org.uk
	Marie Stopes International (reproductive healthcare), www.mariestopes.org.uk
	British Pregnancy Advisory Service, www.bpas.org
	The Menopause Amarant Trust, www.amarantmenopausetrust.org.uk
	Breast Cancer Care, www.breastcancercare.org.uk
Other	Voluntary Euthanasia Society, www.ves.org.uk
	Aviation Health Institute, www.aviation-health.org

Index